GOODBYE POSTPARTUM DEPRESSION AND ANXIETY

SELF-HELP GUIDE FOR MOTHERS TO BALANCE YOUR
EMOTIONS, RESTORE YOUR STRENGTH, AND BUILD
BETTER HABITS

HALEIGH DIOR, M.A.

CONTENTS

INTRODUCTION

The excitement of becoming a mother can often hide the anxious and depressing notions behind a cloud of smoke and mirrors until that fateful day arrives when it all feels real. Something moms don't often discuss and share with parents-to-be is the fact that the journey may be filled with negative and positive emotions combined; sometimes, you won't even know which you feel at the moment. The reason moms don't like sharing how tough motherhood can be is that they feel ashamed or guilty for not resembling the moms on magazine covers and social media blogs. You can almost call it a catch 22 scenario because the guilt prevents moms from setting realistic expectations for other new moms, but this can make motherhood even tougher for the viewers. Even when moms feel like this is nothing like they imagined, they still worry about seeking answers, which sadly makes them more anxious.

Besides, all moms feel nervous and a little blue when their babies arrive, right? That's a complicated question. Maybe you're surrounded by people who seem to have everything under control. You watch other moms juggle the responsibilities of having a newborn with the rest of their lives, which doesn't stand still for anyone. This only makes you start doubting yourself, wondering whether you're just exaggerating the way you feel. Why don't they feel blue? Why do other moms not feel the anxiety crashing down on them? Why on earth can't you feel the magnanimous joy other moms feel during this amazing transition from a woman to a mother? Instead, you feel overwhelmed, exhausted, and constantly fearful that something may go wrong with your baby. You can't even fathom the thoughts running through your mind, but you realize they're there. Alternatively, you may just be feeling low and unsupported in this new journey. Maybe you don't have effective support from family, friends, or even your partner. It may also seem like you're drifting away from your partner.

It's hard to understand how these feelings and thoughts rush into your mind after giving birth. You may even have negative feelings during pregnancy. Having a baby should be the most exciting day of your life. You should love the baby unconditionally from day one, and your motherly instincts should kick in, but they don't. You just feel lost and scared. In another case, you may not even see these feelings creep up on you, but someone has mentioned them. A loved one is trying to help you, but you're not sure if anything's wrong. You feel like you're doing things right. Whatever your experience may be, know one thing; you're not alone! Just under 12% of new moms are overwhelmed enough to develop postpartum depression or PPD (U.S. Department of Health and Human Services, 2018). In a sense, this is positive because you may only have the baby blues, but you can't know this unless you learn to distinguish the differences between the two conditions.

The baby blues is a temporary condition, but postpartum depression isn't. The same applies to postpartum anxiety (PPA). Some moms aren't just feeling the regular new mom nervousness that others experience. Sometimes, it's more than that. To make it worse, along comes mention of a rare condition like postpartum psychosis, but sometimes, moms will just be so anxious about their depression or anxiety symptoms that they *think* they're about to lose control. Knowing the differences between all the mental health conditions you may suffer postpartum is the only way you can move toward an improvement. Playing guessing games and listening to moms who never experienced the conditions may exaggerate your feelings and thoughts.

Moreover, you'll feel too guilty or ashamed to get the help you need. The truth is that PPD, as one example, can stay with you for years without intervention or treatment (Brazier & Nwadike, 2019). Ignoring the problem won't make it go away. Instead, you'll be the person who suffers longer than you need to.

Ask yourself, do you want to feel hopeless, deeply saddened, stressed by things that don't seem to stress other moms, or overwhelmed in any way? Do you want to feel anxious, or do you want to do something to make yourself feel better? Additionally, improving your mental health has vast benefits for your baby and your relationship with your partner and other loved ones. According to experts at the Prenatal Department of the Mayo Clinic, a mom's postpartum anxiety and depression can influence her baby's mental state so much that they could suffer from early mental health disorders (Stygar & Zadroga, 2021). However, having good mental health on your side can promote your baby's development and emotional stability, teaching them lessons for life. Both you and your baby deserve the best of everything. Yes, read that again. *You also deserve the best,* which is something you'll find answers to in this book.

Before anything, you must realize when the baby blues have turned into something more. You'll be better off knowing the differences between the main types of postpartum mental health issues to which you can succumb. Remember that your body has experienced great changes, and so has your mind. Only once you realize where you are now can you do something about it. However, there isn't a reason to panic because the three cornerstones of improving your mental health will be mentioned. You'll learn how to cope with postpartum depression and anxiety so you can flourish as a mom. Even new dads can take some advice to help improve their journeys because they also suffer from changes when a baby arrives. Ultimately, both moms and dads will have the tools they need to help themselves and each other. You'll have the emotional toolkit that protects you from falling into the worst of symptoms.

For some moms, what lies within this book can already change the way you feel, think, and bond with your baby. Indeed, you can develop the relationship you want with your baby and partner, no matter what those connections look like now. These relationships will also move you forward as a family that stands tall against adversities. Suppose your symptoms are still hard to manage, and you still need additional support from professionals, you'll learn about what you can expect and how much control you truly have over your options. There are numerous available treatments should you need to use them, and you're not a weak mother for choosing to give your baby the best. Any improvements you make are signs of determined strength. Shying away from the changes you should make is the only sign of weakness. That doesn't mean you're weak if one treatment doesn't work. It will show weakness if you give up after a failed attempt.

I've had to learn to be tough in the face of challenges myself. That's a hard truth when you consider the fact that I'm a therapist who specializes in postpartum anxiety and depression. The reason I know how hard this journey can be isn't only because I'm trained in the field. It's also because I've been where you are now. I've questioned myself, and I experienced those deeply saddening emotions. At first, it can be confusing to think you can feel both happy and sad at once. Moms with postpartum disorders don't lack a deep love for their babies. They just aren't strong enough to juggle the positive and negative emotions at once. With a little guidance, they can! Even as a therapist, I never dismiss how serious and debilitating postpartum conditions can be for the reason that I was there. I know how it can suck the joy out of motherhood. Becoming a mom is something of which you can be proud. It's a blessing words can't describe.

That gradual or sudden onset of negative feelings and thoughts about motherhood makes you forget how blessed you are to have such a precious baby. Depression and anxiety can cloud your judgment and prevent you from thinking in productive or healthy ways. It doesn't matter how far down this road you've already progressed; you can make a turn for the better. I'm passionate about helping new moms do just that. I believe you deserve the incredibly fulfilling side of motherhood just like anyone else, but it will take a little effort and self-compassion. The strategies I'll share with you have helped many other moms who came to me; some were experiencing a little blueness, but others were in dire situations. Allow me to share these tools with you so your journey can become the most amazing experience you can have in this world. The moment you feel ready to learn it all and find ways to cope with motherhood, dive into the first chapter.

1

POSTPARTUM DEPRESSION: LEARN TO SPOT THE SIGNS

Movies paint the wrong picture about the day we bring our babies home. We see happy moms who appear to have everything together. What these images don't show is the myriad of other emotions new moms feel, whether they're first-time or repeat moms. There's nothing like bringing your baby home, indeed. You can feel a wave of excitement and pride washing over you, but it's also perfectly common for moms to feel overwhelmed and sad. It's okay for them to cry and become confused by their emotions. This is the part we don't see, not even on social media. The lack of real-life examples around us can create a stigma where we think we have to smile broadly and walk tall, even though we feel drained and overwhelmed. This is what prevents new moms from sharing their feelings with other people, not even someone who can help them overcome this unwanted mix of emotions. That's the secret; you *can* overcome the mix.

BABY BLUES

Postpartum blues versus postpartum depression, which one do you think you have? As exciting as it can be to bring a new life into your world, the reality kick can also make most moms take a step back when the baby arrives. Some moms even feel the anticipatory blues before giving birth. A baby is the most gorgeous little blend of you and your partner. They encumber everything good in the world, and their little fingers and toes can melt the stoniest of hearts. That first moment you look down at your baby is otherworldly. He or she causes a flood of emotions, making you feel movements inside yourself you never thought possible. Who could ever imagine that love felt like this? Amidst these incredible notions, you may also feel sneaky negative emotions interfering with the way you want to absorb this beautiful little person. Fear, anxiety, sadness, and even the sudden change in who you are can take you by surprise.

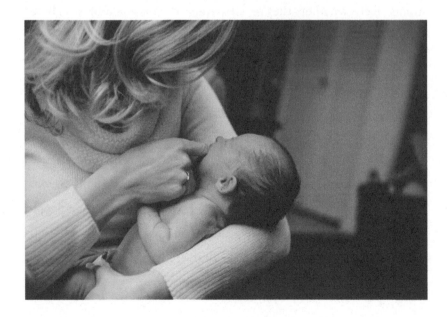

You're already exhausted from giving birth, or you're recovering from a cesarean, but these emotions unfold over and above your tired mind and body. This may just be the first-time you realize that what you expected was nothing like what you feel right now. For some moms, this happens right after birth, and for others, it comes a few days later. A baby is a blessing but also one of the greatest changes you face in life. Any change is bound to make you feel some discomfort. Combine the reality of becoming a mom with the hormonal changes, a completed pregnancy, and giving birth. This transformation often overwhelms moms because it unfolds quickly, leaving some parents feeling like they're not ready, even if they planned everything to a tee. There's an old saying about how we can plan our lives, but life will unravel its own plans. Even the most well-prepared parents are bound to feel a little blue when the baby arrives.

Your wildly unpredictable emotions at this stage are perfectly normal, and this roller coaster is well-known as the baby blues or PPD. As much as movies and social media tell you one thing, know that between 50 and 85% of new moms experience the baby blues (Wisner & Snyder, 2020). Feeling blue doesn't mean you're any less of a mother than someone else. It doesn't mean you have a character flaw and you're about to mess a little person's life up. In contrast, it means you're within the normal range of moms who feel down after bringing a new baby home. You're perfectly human, and your maternal growth isn't non-existent just because you feel a little blue. Before anything, know that you'll be okay, especially if you learn more about the differences between baby blues and PPD. Just the fact that you're seeking knowledge already shows how much you care about yourself and your baby's well-being. Good mothers care enough to learn more.

Baby blues are commonly caused by a change in your routine, hormonal fluctuations, lost sleep, and a temporary self-identity crisis. Humans are habitual creatures, so any changes to your daily routine will naturally disturb your emotional well-being. Your mornings were so methodical until the baby arrived, but you're not even finding time to complete every part of it like you did just before the baby arrived. One quick word of advice here is that you remember to release what isn't within your control. Know that your routine will change, even though you'll try to keep as much consistency as humanly possible. Maybe you can't cook a five-star breakfast tomorrow morning, and that's okay. Find a way to temporarily make faster meals, but try to keep them healthy so that your energy and well-being are balanced. The bottom line is that you must realize in the first few weeks after your baby arrives, things will change.

A secret with babies is that everything will continue changing, but it's up to you to maintain the control you can over things that can be controlled. Sleep deprivation is another reason for the blues. Anyone losing sleep is bound to become emotional. Sleep is one lifeblood that keeps us sane. Sleep disturbances are part of what causes baby blues. Hormonal fluctuations are also to blame. Your body had to produce more estrogen and progesterone during pregnancy to support your baby's development. Suddenly, your levels plummet, which will create emotional fluctuations. The hormonal changes experienced within 24 hours after labor can be similar to premenstrual stress (PMS). Again, hormones are natural changes in your body. You may or may not manage the sudden plunge. Telling from the percentage of moms who suffer from postpartum blues, you're more likely not to cope like a beast with this change, so don't expect it.

The sudden elevation of your mood may also be a result of your body increasingly producing oxytocin and prolactin, which stimulate lactation. This is great for moms who wish to breastfeed. These hormones normally cause positive mood changes, but the confusion in your body caused by hormones pushing your mood to the negative side and back to the positive side can be overwhelmingly exhausting. The self-identity crisis is another common reason for postpartum blues, especially in first-time moms. Before your baby arrived, you were able to make decisions without considering all the responsibilities that come with motherhood. Being a mom is magnificent, but it also comes with a new title, responsibilities, and a loss of freedom. Some new moms struggle with this crisis because they felt in control of their lives and careers, but they quickly became someone entirely different. This realization normally hits after the baby's born.

Most new moms will experience a few baby blue symptoms after bringing their bundles of joy home. Symptoms may include agitation, anxiety, a general overwhelmed sensation, or just feeling off. Waves of sadness may also be accompanied by some tears, but not all of the time. You may experience a change from sadness to joy and vice versa every few minutes, and you could doubt whether you'll look well after your baby. Some moms feel impatient, grumpy, and may even cry over the most ridiculous things. This is your hormones playing ping pong, so it's expected. You may also struggle to eat, concentrate, or make decisions. The baby blues can also make you battle to fall asleep, even when you find some time for shuteye. You may just feel unsettled. Some new moms experience one or two symptoms, and others experience waves of many symptoms.

Postpartum blues may occur right after birth, or they might come four to five days after bringing your baby home. Most women experience these symptoms coming and going for up to two weeks after giving birth. This period is considered normal. Anything that extends past two weeks or the symptoms intensify may be more concerning. The good news is that most moms' symptoms subside within two to three weeks, and they can enjoy their babies and new roles on a broader spectrum. Understand this, a new mom with baby blues also enjoys her baby, but she struggles to find the balance between joy and the blues. It doesn't mean she can't enjoy her baby. Never think you don't love your baby enough. We always need to be consciously aware of what we think about ourselves, knowing how common the baby blues have certainly eased the worries about whether you're doing okay. Additionally, some coping strategies can help you with this potential period.

Accept that what you're feeling is experienced by many new moms, and feel comfortable enough to talk about your emotions with a trusted loved one. There's also no such thing as shame in asking for help around the home and with the baby. Reach out to your loved ones to help yourself rise from the blues, delegate chores to lighten your load. Chances are people will respect you for asking and assist you in ways they can. You can also reach out to a new mom's support group to chat with other moms experiencing the same mood swings and uncertainties. Prioritize your sleep in any way possible, even if you must sleep when your baby sleeps. Otherwise, ask someone at home for help again. Sleep can replenish you in many ways. You can also limit the stressors new moms face, such as having visitors over. Only a new mom knows how exhausting this can be, especially with a newborn. You have a right to say no when you feel tired.

You also need to look after yourself. You can't expect yourself to be the greatest mom who finds joy in this journey if you're falling apart. Eat frequently, and make sure you're getting enough protein and digestible foods. Your body's still healing, so eat food that doesn't make this recovery more challenging with constipation. Get out of the house as well. Ask your partner to help you with the baby while they nap. That way, you can take a slow walk through the park and absorb the beauty of nature. Most important, cut yourself slack. Don't expect yourself to be a supermom by keeping the place shiny and fresh. Of course, you want to live in a clean place, but ask for help again. Hire a cleaner and a cook if you can afford them. Ask a friend to come over and help you with the laundry. Your body and mind are in recovery, so never push yourself harder than you can be expected to move. Letting go a little won't make the world standstill.

The pinnacle of postpartum blues is that you can still function. That's one secret you must consider. If you feel your symptoms gradually subsiding and they don't interfere with your ability to function daily, then you're going to be just fine. If your symptoms intensify and you feel unable to look after yourself and your baby, then you may be heading to postpartum depression. Ask yourself three questions to determine the possibility of you developing PPD.

Question one is how often do you feel sad? Once a day may not be worrisome, but feeling sad or crying most of the day indicates that you may be developing PPD.

Question two is how long does your sadness last? Hormonal fluctuations can cause sudden sadness bouts that last a few minutes or even half an hour. However, sadness that seems to follow you the whole day or for a few days or weeks is likely PPD.

Question three is how intense you would say your sadness feels? Regular hormonal fluctuations may bring sadness that resembles finding out your favorite store closed down. It comes and goes, and it may intensify slightly. However, sadness related to PPD can feel like grief. It can feel like you've lost something or someone so dear that it overwhelms you.

If you suspect PPD, I implore that you keep learning more about the disorder because it's entirely manageable. Don't feel alone, and never allow a temporary change in your moods and emotional well-being to deter you from the joyous journey you deserve. Reach out to a therapist, speak to them about medication safe to use while breastfeeding if you're doing that, and apply some simple changes to your routine so that you can smile broadly and genuinely. But first, learn how PPD looks and feels.

POSTPARTUM DEPRESSION

When the blues turn into depression, seeking some guidance and coping mechanisms can make a huge difference for you and your baby. According to research conducted by the Centers for Disease

Control and Prevention (CDC), postpartum depression only affects one in nine new moms (Ko et al., 2017). Honestly, we'd love to see that number come down even further, but knowing PPD is less common than the baby blues can give you a little peace of mind. If you're one of the new moms who fall into this number, fear not; you can still overcome it. Even though your body and mind have experienced massive changes during pregnancy and birth, motherhood is not characterized by feeling hopeless, empty, and sad most of the time. PPD is unlike the baby blues. It's more serious, and it can affect your brain and the way it functions, which may change your behavior and even your physical health.

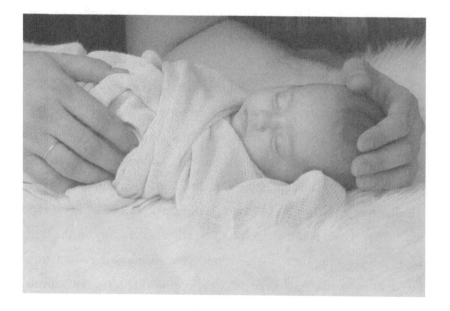

You and your baby deserve better than feeling hopeless or empty most of the time. PPD can be caused by the same hormonal factors as the baby blues, but new moms also tend to have concerns about the recovery after giving birth. Your body has transformed in many physical ways, and you might be worried about losing the baby weight. Even something as simple as body image insecurities can contribute to PPD. You may fear whether you're still attractive to your partner. Our relationships are the glue that holds us together so that this contribution can create depressive symptoms. Stress is another factor that contributes to your likelihood of developing PPD. Caring for a newborn isn't a walk in the park due to the loss of sleep, having to feed your baby on demand, and the change of identity you're experiencing. Some stress is expected during this transitional time, so don't be hard on yourself.

The symptoms of PPD are similar to the baby blues, but they're more aggressive and last longer. You may feel restless, angry, and irritable, and you'll experience excessive crying bouts. Sometimes, you won't even know why you're crying. Your appetite and energy levels will be low, and you'll look for reasons to sleep more and more. There will be a feeling of disconnection from your life, almost as though you're living in third-person mode. You may suffer from insomnia, nightmares, or even obsessively racing and frightening thoughts. You'll experience low self-esteem, feeling like you can't be a good mother. You may feel worthless, guilty, and anxious most of the time. More severe symptoms may include you withdrawing from your loved ones, feeling an urge to escape your life or even suicidal ideations. The more severe symptoms aren't part of the baby blues.

The severe symptoms may also include you not being able to care for yourself or your newborn. You may struggle to bond with your bundle of joy, and thoughts of self-harm or harming your baby may enter your mind. Firstly, if you think of harming yourself or your baby, even just for a passing moment, please contact the Suicide Prevention Hotline on **1-800-273-8255** or visit your nearest emergency room immediately. No one will judge you for seeking help. It's the bravest thing you can do when harmful thoughts come into your mind. Seeking help during this time is a sign that you're not prepared to allow the thoughts to control you. Reaching out will only prove that you're motivated to control your thoughts. Also, you can contact your healthcare provider if your next check-up is far away and you feel like you have PPD. Talking to them is another brave step that shows how committed you are to being the best mother.

If you find yourself just wishing that you weren't alive, it also helps to reach out to someone who can help you, even if you just need a moment to absorb nature in the park while your partner watches the baby. Withdrawing from your loved ones can also be quite concerning because you need social support. Have you ever heard that a whole village is needed to raise a child? Indeed, your loved ones can be your village. If you can't speak to them, call a professional to help you cope with the urge to withdraw from loved ones. One truth we forget in life is that there's always a way forward. If you feel like you can't rely on the people around you, or you feel disconnected from your partner, you can always approach your doctor to find support where you'll feel more comfortable until you can open up to your loved ones. You can also use the *Edinburgh Postnatal Depression Scale* to see whether you need help if you're afraid of reaching out first. A score above 13 would indicate PPD. You can find the scale at:

www.helpguide.org/wp-content/uploads/edinburghscale.pdf

PPD is also unlike the baby blues in that it can start gradually within the first year of your baby's life. You may feel excited and capable for the first three months before you start feeling the urge to cry for reasons you don't even know. The stress of taking care of your new baby, your hormone changes, and even the grief of losing your self-identity is known to contribute to the possibility of developing PPD. However, some new moms are at a greater risk of developing it. The University of Pittsburgh researched the potential identifiers that could more easily predispose someone to PPD, and the results were published in *Clinical Obstetrics and Gynecology* (Sit & Wisner, 2009). A few risk factors were mentioned in the review. Firstly, women younger than 20 are more likely to suffer from PPD. This may be due to them losing their self-identity at such a young age. It may also be due to them feeling the need to be perfect mothers.

Other risk factors include whether you have bipolar disorder or a history of depression, and a family history of either condition will also increase your risk of developing PPD. Another risk factor is when new moms don't have support from their loved ones and social groups. PPD can also develop easier in someone who was depressed during pregnancy or had difficulties with the pregnancy. An unplanned pregnancy could also lead to PPD, and so can breastfeeding challenges. Additionally, alcoholism and a history of addictive behaviors can also cause PPD after birth. Finally, a big risk factor in the review was when new moms give birth to a baby with special needs. This only adds to their stress. It doesn't mean they can't be the best mom and enjoy the journey, but special needs babies naturally come with a little added stress and responsibility. It's quite natural to feel overwhelmed with a special needs baby.

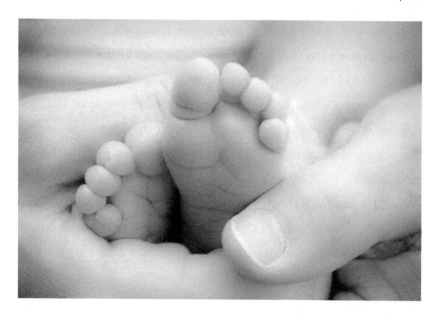

If you think you're suffering from PPD, or you realize you're at greater risk, reach out to someone. As a therapist and mom, I intend to give you the tools to manage your depression, but you can also seek therapy or medication to add to this toolkit, which we'll discuss in Chapter 7. New moms certainly have a lot on their plates, but people forget or dismiss the idea that dads can also suffer from PPD. The causes aren't well-known, but the risk factors are increased when a mom suffers from PPD, or a dad previously suffered from depression or bipolar disorder. It's important for dads to also look after their mental health when a new baby arrives. Dads don't see the PPD sneaking up on them as easily because it happens gradually. Their symptoms will mirror those of a mother. Even though PPD in dads is rarer than in moms, the condition is known to exist and has a name—paternal postpartum depression (Mayo Clinic Staff, 2018).

Whether you, your partner or both of you have PPD, consider adding coping strategies to your arsenal so you can both be the great parents you're bound to be. The best first step you can take toward overcoming depression in any form is to accept that you feel depressed. Accepting a truth opens doors to changing it. Moreover, the coping strategies you'll learn in this book and from healthcare professionals will help you maintain your mental health for years to come. It's not just about coping with a newborn. It's also about maintaining a good state of mental health for yourself and your loved ones for life so that you all have the best experience and closest bonds you can achieve.

POSTPARTUM PSYCHOSIS

This is a condition we hardly hear about, and that's due to it being so rare. According to the U.S. Department of Health and Human Services, postpartum psychosis only develops in four out of every 1000 women (2018). It's also an emergency mental health transition that requires urgent medical attention. This condition will develop within the first two weeks after your newborn comes home. Your risk of developing it will increase if you have bipolar or schizoaffective disorder, the latter of which is a combination of mood disorder and schizophrenia. Having either one of these disorders is already a reason to discuss it with your doctor before giving birth. You may be helped before the condition can develop after your baby arrives. However, the rarity of the disorder gives you peace of mind, especially if you don't have those pre-existing conditions. If you do, and you develop postpartum psychosis, please seek immediate medical assistance.

Again, you won't be judged. Seeking assistance is a sign of you wanting to be the best for yourself and your baby. Healthcare professionals spend years learning how to help you, so allow them to put their studies to practice. The symptoms are also intense, so even your loved ones may notice that you need emergency care. Some symptoms include hallucinations, delusions, and excessive mood swings. Hallucinations are when you hear and see things that aren't really there. You may feel crawling under your skin, or you might hear your baby crying when they're sleeping. Delusions are the unrealistic beliefs we have, even in the face of evidence. For example, you may start believing that your baby will come to harm if they don't start eating more food, even though experts agree that a newborn must be fed on demand until they're satisfied. Even visiting the doctor who tells you how well your baby's doing might not change your belief.

The excessive mood swings may include moments of manic depression and euphoria with only minutes between them. You may laugh one moment and cry another. Paranoia is another common symptom of postpartum psychosis. You might start thinking someone is out to hurt your baby when there's no evidence to support it. Your paranoia may be that someone wants to take your baby away or harm you. Reckless behavior is another sign. Mental confusion and excessive restlessness can also be symptoms, and you may feel disorientated or have obsessive thoughts about your baby. Unusual behavior, suicidal thoughts, and thoughts of harming your baby are severe symptoms that need **immediate medical attention**. You won't feel like this forever, so reaching out is the best way to keep you, your baby, and your partner safe and happy.

If you are a partner who notices psychotic symptoms, please don't worry about what your partner will and won't think about; *get them some help*. They'll appreciate the sentiment once they feel normal again, which *will* happen. The possibility of postpartum psychosis may be frightening, but don't let it deter you from enjoying your new journey. Consider the risk factors, and know when to seek help. Otherwise, allow the baby blues to pass or learn coping strategies to elevate your mental health if you suffer from PPD, but most of all, know that the journey will become more enjoyable than you can imagine. Knowledge and awareness will prevent it from being anything else.

2

POSTPARTUM ANXIETY: THE SYMPTOMS

Talking about baby blues is quite common; however, postpartum anxiety is less commonly discussed, even though it may be more prevalent in new moms. Just like PPD, postpartum anxiety can also blend in with the regular excitement new parents feel when a baby comes home. Anxiety is a general fear that something is about to go wrong, so it's understandable that new parents may feel nervous to some extent, especially first-time parents. Newborns can be unpredictable. Much of what they do is enough to make you see the world through new eyes, but they can also make you nervous when those unexpected experiences occur. For new parents, a newborn may be full of unexpected occurrences, so you must know what PPA looks and feels like if you want to enjoy your parenting journey.

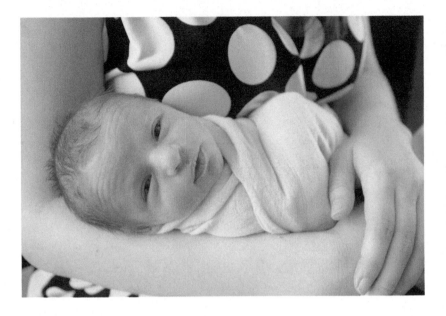

POSTPARTUM ANXIETY BASICS

Let's talk about Megan for a moment. She just became a new mom for the first-time. Megan has friends and relatives, but they're all in other states due to her partner taking a new job in Boston. The idea of a new life is exciting for Megan and Jack, and the baby's arrival just adds to the list of unknowns. Sometimes, unknowns can be exciting, but we don't realize that they naturally cause anxiety. To make it worse, Megan is stuck at home with her newborn. She has no friends or loved ones nearby to help her. Jack is relentlessly trying to make an impression with his new job, so he's also not around much. Megan has never been a mom until the day her baby came home. She attended prenatal classes back in Mississippi, and she read many books about what she must do when the baby arrives. The only problem is that she's having these overwhelming thoughts, and she thinks they're normal. In some cases, they are normal and expected, but Megan's case is slightly different.

Megan's joy quickly turns into fear as she holds her baby near her nipple. She can't get the little one to latch on properly, and the baby cries endlessly. She doesn't know how to get her baby fed, and she turns to a bottle. It doesn't make much of a difference as her baby continues crying. What Megan doesn't realize is that she has a colic baby. After some quick reading, she finally understands colic babies, or so she thinks. Now, she fears holding the baby over the length of her arm to administer the movements that could help her baby release gas. What if her baby falls? What if she drops her baby? What if her baby chokes? She has 100 thoughts flashing through her mind. She thinks she's about to harm her baby. What does Megan do? She leaves the baby crying because she's too afraid to help him. She doesn't trust herself. She can only see herself hurting the baby, even though she doesn't intend to.

Megan's thoughts make her cringe, but she can't help having them. What Megan's story teaches us is that her anxiety prevented her from trying to help her baby. It doesn't help that Megan didn't have support around her. Her anxiety was compounded by the move to a new state, having no relatives around for support, not knowing what her future holds with her partner's new job, and now, the baby arrives. New moms who fear hurting their babies are suffering from a form of general anxiety disorder that commonly follows having a baby. Dealing with this anxiety is simple and may only require some education about PPA, but leaving the problem for additional fear of being seen as a bad mother only compounds the effects more.

Additionally, Megan's little one is also struggling because she's too afraid to do what she must do. Fortunately, colic babies are common, and it's something they'll outgrow.

However, some new moms will fear bathing their babies because they have thoughts of drowning them. The thoughts are in no way intentional, and they can never see themselves doing it, but the thoughts happen anyway. A mom with PPA will never intentionally harm her baby, and one differentiating sign between PPA and postpartum psychosis is that a mom will feel bad for even thinking that way. Feeling bad about it doesn't remove the thoughts, though. Moms need to address the fears, or they won't overcome them. PPA isn't all about compounding fears, either. Sometimes, a new mom or dad can just feel a little overwhelmed with a new baby. They might fear not being a good mom or dad, or they may think about how the baby can fall when they change their diapers. How will they afford all the baby supplies in this new time of uncertainty? Will dad still have a job six months from now? Will mom still have her investment income?

The biggest challenge with PPA is that severe symptoms may seem like postpartum psychosis, but the difference is that you'll be repulsed by your thoughts with PPA. The screening for PPA is also complex. The same test shared in Chapter 1 can also screen for symptoms of anxiety. In some cases, symptoms from PPA and PPD may overlap, which also creates confusion. However, just as baby blues are common, anxious feelings are also natural for new moms. Research published in the *Journal of Affective Disorders* followed more than 300 new moms to determine the prevalence of PPA versus PPD over three months postnatal (Fairbrother et al., 2016). All the moms were screened for both disorders right after childbirth, and those who showed signs of either disorder were screened again at three months after childbirth. The moms who didn't screen for symptoms were used as a control group.

The prevalence of PPD at the three-month check-up was 4.8% among moms who showed signs after childbirth and 3.9% among the control group moms. More surprisingly, 17.1% of moms who showed symptoms of mood disorders after childbirth were showing PPA symptoms three months later, and 15.8% of the control group moms showed anxiety symptoms, respectively. The most interesting result found in the research was that anxiety symptoms were more common than depression symptoms among these first-time mothers. Some risk factors were also noted in the paper. Women are more likely to suffer from PPA than men, and a family history of anxiety or depression also increases the new mom's risk. PPA might be harder to pinpoint in new moms, and better screening may be necessary, but PPA may be more common than PPD. Keep in mind that the two may still overlap in symptoms.

Other risk factors for developing PPA are having a history of eating disorders, being diagnosed with obsessive-compulsive disorder (OCD), and if you had previous troubles with pregnancy and childbirth. Maybe you lost your first baby, which certainly makes you more anxious about the new baby. Even pregnancy complications may cause higher anxiety levels. Some women who suffer from weepiness and extreme agitation during PMS can also be at greater risk for PPA. You may just be someone who easily worries about the well-being of others, which is known as personality type A. There's nothing wrong with being a sensitive person as long as it doesn't affect your life. Anxiety is a natural reaction in your body, which may also follow those hormonal fluctuations. Pregnant and new moms hate hearing that their hormones are all over the place again, but keep in mind that the fluctuations are scientifically responsible for the changes.

You're allowed to feel the fluctuations as long as you notice what's normal and what isn't. Just the stress of having a baby and keeping them safe can also send your hormones all over the place. Stress results in hormonal changes in your body. Cortisol and adrenaline are hormones, and having them in your body for prolonged periods naturally leads to anxiety; other common reasons for having PPA include societal expectations. All these moms prance around and pretend as though having a newborn is all smiles and giggles. Suddenly, you think you have to be perfect. You must be happy at all times. People only display what they want others to see, so don't believe that every newborn is a dream. Newborns at least cause nervousness. Know that comparing yourself and your baby to other moms based on societal expectations is a flawed plan. It will only lead you to PPA. Your expectations are what matters.

Educate yourself about what can go wrong, as you're doing now, but also educate yourself about the good things you can expect. Newborns don't only come with nervous moments. They also bring moments where cherished memories are made. Look at both sides of a coin to know its true value. Finally, the changes in your interpersonal and intimate relationships after giving birth can also make you anxious.

Maybe your partner seems distant, so you worry about them leaving you for someone else. You don't think you're attractive anymore, so your fears about losing your partner grow. Understand that your partner may also be dealing with the changes to the family dynamics, so working together toward a mutually beneficial outcome can even expand your relationship to new levels. However, fears surrounding relationships are a common cause of PPA.

You might even fear losing a friend because they don't seem to like babies. Indeed, you get some people who don't like babies. Can you believe it? In contrast, you might have a friend who seems too lovable with your baby, and you think that they're about to snatch your little one and run away. Fear doesn't always know logic, so don't be surprised about what makes you anxious. Anxiety on some level is adaptive, and it's something you can be proud of, knowing that you're concerned about your baby's well-being. Anxiety is merely a natural consequence of a desire to protect your baby, and that already makes you a good mom. Worrying about your baby's safety, and worrying about whether you'll be able to give your baby what they need, bridges the gap between a mom who doesn't care or behaves recklessly and a mom who cares enough to feel anxious. For many new moms, their anxieties create an inner chatter that only sounds like noise, and they brush it off.

For example, maybe you fear hurting your baby's little wrist when you dress them. This is a rational fear, and all it does is increase your attention to prevent it from happening. You may fear that you can't help your baby develop the skills they need, so you learn about games you can play with them to promote their development. There's nothing wrong with that. You might worry about your baby crying because they're hungry, so you feed them. Again, nothing's wrong here. However, your anxiety can be greater and irrational enough to prevent you from enjoying motherhood. You may experience some symptoms of depression, such as having a lack of interest in your baby or feeling sad all of the time, but PPA commonly manifests as worries. It seems like a loss of balance between rational and irrational thoughts, but PPD is more of a loss of heart.

Your anxiety may even start before you give birth. Between 25 and 35% of new moms develop PPA before birth (Collno & Fabian-Weber, 2020). It can also develop right after birth, within the first year, after a stressful life event, or when you wean your baby. Symptoms may include a lasting sense of doom or dread, and you'll have excessive thoughts about your baby's safety and development. You may constantly feel like something bad is about to happen, or you may experience racing thoughts. Your desire to be the best parent will become overbearing and feel more like a burden than a blessing. You may feel agitated and suffer from insomnia or other sleep disturbances. You might experience unexplained and frequent nausea, dizziness, chills, hot flashes, or jitters. You'll also notice a change in your heartbeat and breathing, which may lead to panic attacks. Your worries won't easily be appeased, and you'll likely feel exhausted more than usual.

Concentration will be but a dream, and any of these symptoms will be far more intense than that of a normal new mom who merely worries about simple things. Again, worry is a certainty, but consider whether your worries are affecting your ability to function and be the best you can be. And no, that doesn't mean perfection. It means you're capable of addressing your and your baby's needs. PPA also tends to manifest illogically. Your fears may have no evidence to support them, and they may persist longer than expected. Moreover, if you suffer from moments of panic and physical manifestations like a rapid heart rate, you're probably experiencing PPA. If you feel like your anxiety is standing in the way of addressing your or your baby's needs, then you may be too anxious.

TWO MAIN TYPES

Postpartum anxiety can be categorized into two subtypes. The first type of PPA is called postpartum panic disorder. The second type of PPA is called postpartum obsessive-compulsive disorder (OCD). Keep in mind that any postpartum disorders must be diagnosed by a medical professional. You can know what to look out for, but only a doctor can diagnose you. That means a relative also can't tell you that you're just nervous like every other new mom unless they have a medical degree.

Postpartum Panic Disorder

This type of PPA is estimated to affect up to 10% of new moms (Carberg & Langdon, 2016). However, it's also suspected that many cases go undiagnosed due to stigma and societal influence, much like a relative telling you that nervousness is normal. Panic disorders cause physiological, mental, and emotional distress in your body and mind. They should never be ignored if you suspect them.

Risk factors for developing postpartum panic disorder include:

- Thyroid dysfunctions
- Hormonal changes
- Past experiences with panic and anxiety disorders
- A lack of sleep
- Poor nutrition
- Traumatic or challenging childbirth

Some new moms may relive the trauma they experienced during childbirth. Having no support financially or from your loved ones can also compound the effects of panic disorders. Our bodies are designed to respond to anything that threatens our well-being, even if we aren't genuinely in danger.

The biological changes in your body and mind can cascade into physical symptoms because the part of your brain responsible for your stress response doesn't know the difference between logical and illogical thoughts. Fears can conjure irrational thinking patterns that cause your body to respond to what it perceives as a threat. The stress hormones increase your blood pressure and heart rate to make you alert and ready for action. For new moms, this biological response can lead to panic attacks. The symptoms that lead to physical changes may come gradually or suddenly, the former being more concerning because you don't always notice them until you're about to have a panic attack. Normal new mom nervousness doesn't lead to panic attacks. That's only due to a panic disorder, which is a mental health problem that could steal the joy from your journey. The three main fears moms with panic disorder face are the fear of death, the fear of losing control, and the fear of losing their minds.

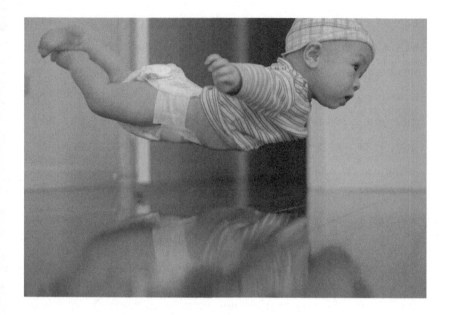

The symptoms that may gradually grab hold of you include an inability to remember things or concentrate. You may struggle to complete tasks, be easily distracted, and find it hard to make decisions. You might feel edgy and unable to relax, and you could struggle with fatigue, insomnia, and a lost appetite. An impending sense of dread may follow you for prolonged times, even if you don't know what you dread. You'll feel agitated and uninterested in going outside. Agoraphobia or the fear of open and public spaces is a sign of postpartum panic disorder. You may even avoid events and commitments because you're afraid something bad will happen. More concerning, you may experience panic attacks and suicidal thoughts. Panic attacks are classified as the presence of four or more of the symptoms related to them. Panic attacks cause shortness of breath, chest pain or pressure, suffocating sensations, and excessive sweating.

Panic attacks may also include hot flashes, heart palpitations, extreme chills, trembling, and a tingling sensation in your arms or legs. You may become lightheaded or feel like you're about to faint. Your stomach will be upset, and you'll feel disconnected from the world while you experience a panic attack. You may even feel impending doom or thoughts of lingering death overwhelm you. Panic attacks are quite serious, and they can even feel like heart attacks. These are the physiological changes instigated by your stress hormones. However, a panic attack only lasts 20 to 30 minutes in most cases. It shouldn't go longer than an hour. The intensity of a panic attack will also increase around 10 minutes into the response.

The best way for you to overcome postpartum panic disorder is by learning how to recognize the symptoms and apply tools to help you defeat them. Seeking help from a therapist or taking prescribed medicine to soothe your anxiety can also help, but managing anxiety disorders is an ongoing process. Managing any mental health condition should be treated as an ongoing practice.

Postpartum Obsessive-Compulsive Disorder

Postpartum OCD is what Megan was experiencing. She was so obsessed with her baby's well-being and safety that it prevented her from doing what she had to. Obsession never leads to perfection. Quite the opposite, it can lead to procrastination or an inability to act. Postpartum OCD affects between three and five percent of new moms (Brusie & Snyder, 2020). The causes are also not definitive, but it's most probable that women who suffered from OCD before or during pregnancy will also express the symptoms after giving birth. Showing symptoms of OCD during pregnancy is a perinatal disorder. Stress is a major trigger for anyone with OCD, so new moms bringing a baby home is a trigger for postpartum OCD. Your hormones may also interfere with your serotonin and other neurotransmitter functions, which also triggers it.

Nervousness remains a normal part of being a new mom. Determining whether you may have postpartum OCD or regular nervousness is a matter of considering how much it consumes your thoughts and how it affects your ability to function. If you feel that your fears and thoughts are taking control of your life, then postpartum OCD might be an issue you must overcome. Moms with OCD will obsess over their baby's health, safety, and development to an extent where they end up in Megan's situation. They won't likely have compulsive behaviors, but some new moms express compulsivity. For example, a mom with postpartum OCD who also expresses compulsiveness may constantly visit her doctor for fears that her baby's unwell. She may also pray excessively or have someone on speed dial to seek reassurance before she does anything with her baby.

She won't rely on her intuitiveness or motherly instincts. Indeed, we can never be too careful with our babies, but we also can't allow our compulsiveness or obsessiveness to prevent us from actually caring for ourselves and our babies. The obsessive side of this disorder may present as thoughts about the baby being harmed, whether a mom thinks she will accidentally harm the baby or her lack of knowledge and experience will do it. Some symptoms of postpartum OCD include worrying about the baby dying from sudden infant death syndrome (SIDS). On a side note, which hopefully eases your fears about something like SIDS, only 35 of 100,000 babies succumb to this tragedy (Taylor, 2020). The risk of SIDS is minimal, so even though it's a genuine concern, albeit it's also aggravated by baby product warning labels, the chances of your baby coming to harm remain *minute*. Anyway, other fears also happen with OCD.

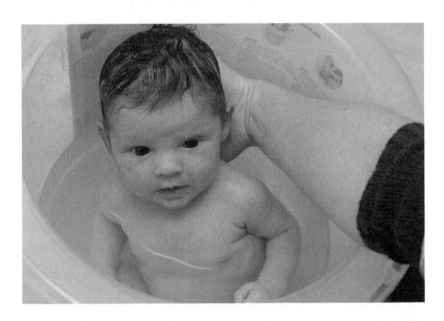

You may fear your baby falling, you dropping them, their heads going under the water in a bath, or finding them unresponsive. You may even imagine yourself placing the baby in ridiculous places like the microwave, which in all seriousness, is unlikely. Additionally, you may picture yourself shaking your baby, and you'll feel absolutely repulsed by the thought afterward. Remember that your ability to feel repulsed and your awareness of how grotesque these fears sound are signs that you're not suffering from postpartum psychosis. You more likely have postpartum OCD. You can always discuss your symptoms with a mental healthcare professional if you still feel worried about your thoughts. No harm can come from seeking a professional opinion. Consider whether you obsess over your baby's safety and well-being. If so, it wouldn't hurt to get a diagnosis. That way, you can use the tools in this book and seek professional mental health guidance if you want to overcome this condition. Postpartum OCD is something you may have to learn to manage for years.

A POSITIVE OUTLOOK

Any mental health challenge we face is unpredictable and has no time limits. Wanting to know how long your symptoms may last is normal, but is there a magic end date for you to suddenly feel better? Every woman experiences PPA and PPD at their own pace, and many variables can contribute to how long you need to mentally care for yourself. The first reason it's a challenge to determine an end date is that both conditions aren't normally researched past the first year after your baby arrives. We know that they can start before or within the first year of your baby's life, but we aren't certain about how it affects women beyond this. According to a small study mentioned in *The Telegraph*, postpartum depression strikes many women when their toddlers turn four (Smith, 2014). Research is showing that PPD and PPA have no definitive onset or resolution time.

Other variables that could influence your resolution include how severe your condition became, whether you have a history of mental health disorders, and how long you waited to reach out. More variables include how much support you have among loved ones, the environment you're in, and how dedicated you are to practicing self-care and professional improvement exercises. If your condition is severe, you may require medication, therapy, and self-care habits to reinforce a positive outcome. You may also need to maintain your improved mental state once you reach it. Parenthood comes with many challenges, so continuing your self-care practices at home will help you become resilient against the disorders. It's also common for your symptoms to come and go while your children grow up. Being the epicenter of improved mental well-being can help not only you but your children can thrive from your example.

The upcoming chapters are about to teach you how to improve your mental health by practicing simple self-care habits. Your lifestyle provides better control over your mental health, and if you feel like it's not enough, you can always reach out to a therapist or consider medication. The more tools you add to your arsenal, the better your chances of success will be. The positive truth of your condition is that it *can* be treated, whether you have PPD or PPA. You *can* and *will* get better through self-care, support, and in some cases, therapy and medication. The secret to defeating PPA and PPD is that you never stop practicing what you learn in the next three chapters. It's the foundation of what makes your mental state peaceful and manageable.

3

PHYSICAL SELF-CARE: EXERCISE, DIET, AND SLEEP

New moms think they must put their needs aside for their babies. This fallacy is what leads to many moms struggling on this journey. The key is that you have to care for yourself just as much as your baby. Your body needs to have the energy and stamina to cope with a newborn. What you do for your body and physical health will give you the means to provide the best for your baby. You can't provide what you don't possess. It's easy to allow your physical health to fall by the wayside when a baby arrives, and having PPD or PPA can only make it more challenging to care for yourself. Ensuring that you address the three elements of your physical well-being will make motherhood a whole lot simpler. These elements also reduce the effects of PPA and PPD.

ELEMENT ONE: EXERCISE

Symptoms of depression have long been known to decline with physical activity, so it was also researched regarding PPD. A systematic review of 12 different studies was published in *Birth* (Poyatos-León et al., 2017). The criteria included new moms who measured high on PPD scales compared to a control group of moms who never measured high enough or reported any symptoms. The conclusion of all 12 studies supported the idea that physical activity can reduce the symptoms of PPD. The analysis also focused on which types of exercise routines were used in the studies and whether an improved overall psychological well-being was achieved. The range of exercise routines used were pram walking, yoga, cardiovascular workouts, and light stretching. Improved psychological well-being was also shared among the studies. Exercise is the first element that could improve your psychological health and reduce the symptoms of PPD, in particular.

Exercise is an important part of your recovery and self-care. It's a new habit you should practice as part of your lifestyle going forward. One of the main reasons exercise works against PPD is that it activates the release of endorphins in the brain. Endorphins are natural drugs that don't come with side effects. Some people may compare endorphins to morphine. They can attach themselves to the receptors on your neurons, which are your brain cells, and this reduces pain. Another endorphin is called dopamine, and it's known as a natural antidepressant. It can halt the spread of stress hormones, and it can boost your positive feelings. Dopamine is also part of the reward system, so it increases feelings of pleasure.

Serotonin is another hormone released, and it's most famously known for regulating all the other hormones in your body and reproductive system, which includes the stress hormones. Helping your body release endorphins is the most natural way to control your moods by keeping yourself physically healthy. Exercise also promotes better sleep, strengthens your abdominal and pelvic muscles, and gives you a boost of energy to manage your baby's needs better. You only have so much energy after giving birth and the weeks that follow, so help yourself cope with this time by flooding yourself with hormones that promote better energy. You don't need to live in the gym, either. Exercising or staying physically active for 20 to 30 minutes daily can do the trick.

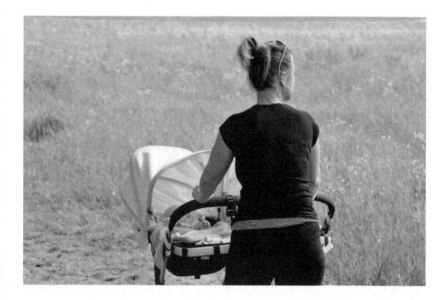

When can you start exercising? Exercise after a normal vaginal birth with no complications can be initiated once you feel comfortable, albeit the regular waiting period is around six weeks. Gentle exercises like walking, pelvic or tummy exercises, Kegels, and gentle stretches are fine if you feel fit enough. The six-week postpartum check-up is a good time to discuss exercise with your doctor. You might even start your gentle routines with five-minute stints. Women who were active before and during pregnancy may be able to return to a gradual routine earlier. However, it's always best to discuss any exercise plans with a doctor. Listen to your body, watch for red flags that caution against exercise, and go at a pace that makes you comfortable. You can begin modified and gentle exercises right after birth if your doctor says it's fine, you have no warning symptoms, and you had a regular vaginal birth without complications. Increase your intensity gradually over the first few weeks.

If you experienced vaginal tearing during childbirth, you need two to three weeks to recover from a third- or fourth-degree tear before you consider exercising. Your doctor may encourage walking or upper body exercises. If you had a cesarean, you'll most likely have to wait for the six-week check-up. However, you should begin walking as soon as you can after a cesarean. This promotes better circulation and prevents blood clots. It can also help you pass gas more easily. High-intensity exercise depends on variables. If you were sedentary before giving birth, you shouldn't be running marathons or doing CrossFit just because you want to shake the baby weight. Highly active exercisers who continued their CrossFit, running, jogging, cycling, and interval training before and during pregnancy until they weren't comfortable anymore may still be able to return to a modified version of the higher intensity workouts about four weeks after birth.

However, it doesn't matter how fit you were before childbirth; always listen to your body and stop when you see red flags. It also helps to know what you can expect when you start exercising. Your body isn't what it was for a few weeks and months after childbirth. Your core abdominal muscles and lower back may not be as strong as they were before childbirth. Your joints and ligaments become more flexible and sensitive during pregnancy, and this will take some time to strengthen again. Stretching or twisting too abruptly could lead to injuries.

Additionally, your old sports bra won't fit now. Measure yourself professionally for a new one if you can afford it. The bottom line is that you should also not expect your body to respond the same way to exercise as it once did, even if you were highly active before.

Another tip for exercising after birth applies to new moms who breastfeed. The best way to approach this is by feeding your baby before going for a jog or walk. This makes your breasts more comfortable if they bounce around. Your breastmilk may also cause a reaction from your baby after exercising because it becomes more acidic. This is only temporary, so don't let it trouble you. It can't harm your baby. It may just taste different. Breastfeeding before exercising is the best answer, but you can still exercise when you choose to breastfeed a baby.

The red flags are the signs you should stop exercising and speak to your doctor. Sometimes, your body just isn't ready when you think it is. You should stop exercising and visit your doctor for advice if you start bleeding after your lochia has vanished. Lochia is the blood, mucus, and discharge that follows birth. This normally lasts around six weeks, albeit some moms have it a little longer or shorter. It's a natural process after birth. You'll have lochia after any type of birth. If you notice it comes back, or it changes suddenly when you exercise, stop your routine and stick to walking while you follow your doctor's advice. Besides, the maternity pads used during this phase don't make exercise easy anyway. You'll be far more comfortable once you lose those maternity boats.

Other red flags that require a halt on exercise include abdominal or vaginal pain and leakage of other fluids like feces or urine. Your nether regions are still recovering, so these signs may indicate that your body wasn't ready to exercise yet. You should also be conscious of any pressure in your vaginal region or reproductive organs because this may indicate a prolapse, which is when the organs come down the vaginal canal. Remember that all the muscles in this region are stretched and exhausted. They need enough time to recover. Any of these red flag signs encourage a halt until your body is genuinely ready for a workout.

Postpartum Exercise Ideas

New moms may feel out of place with their changing and recovering bodies, but there are some great options to try postpartum. Join a postnatal exercise group led by a qualified instructor who also knows your body's limits. Additionally, most of them allow you to bring your baby along, making it double as a bonding exercise. You may even use your baby's stroller or buggy to help in certain routines. Postnatal yoga classes can also offer the same benefits while showing you how you can safely stretch while including your baby in the routine. Always make sure your instructor is a postnatal expert, and don't forget to tell them you've just had a baby. It can be difficult to take your baby to postnatal yoga before they have control over their little bobbling necks. The instructor may even recommend that your baby only becomes part of your workouts once they can support their necks.

You can also build physical workouts into your regular routine by taking the stairs instead of an elevator. Walk to the supermarket instead of driving if it's close. Play active games with your older children, or do stroller walks. Push your stroller briskly as you walk, but keep your back straight and arms bent. Your elbows should make a right angle if your stroller's handles are at the right height. You can also practice knee-bending instead of relying on your waist or back when you pick things up. If you're picking up heavy objects, hold them close to your body while you keep your spine straight and your knees bent outward.

Furthermore, you can look for postnatal exercise videos online, including gentle yoga stretches. Swimming is a gentle and low-impact exercise to get all your muscles working. Just be sure that your postpartum bleeding has stopped for at least seven days before you swim, and bring someone along who can watch the baby so you can do a few gentle laps.

Strengthening your pelvic floor after birth is recommended. It results in improved sensations when you become intimate again, but it will also help you recover faster from unstable pelvic, back, and stomach muscles that could lead to leaky syndrome after having a baby. New moms are particularly embarrassed by the incontinence that comes from weak muscles in their lower bodies. Strengthening the muscles will also help to get your joints back in shape, so you don't have lower back problems at a later stage. To make it sound even more tempting, pelvic, lower back, and stomach muscle exercises can be practiced in the first six weeks as soon as you feel comfortable. Keep an eye out for those red flags, but you should be good to go, especially with Kegels and gentle workouts. Find postpartum videos online, or you can use these gentle approaches:

Kegels are great for strengthening your pelvic floor. You can do them anywhere and anytime. Sit with your back straight while you pull your muscles in your vagina tighter. Imagine you're holding a wee, and then release the hold. Repeat Kegels 20 times, three times a day.

A lateral pelvic tilt also strengthens your muscles. Get down on all fours on a gentle but firm surface. Keep your back straight as you move one leg back to straighten it. This tilts your body slightly. Bring it down and tilt the other side. Only hold each tilt as long as you find it comfortable, and don't stretch your leg too far out to cause a strain.

Gentle ab curls are also safe as long as you don't push past your comfort zone. Lie comfortably flat on your back while keeping your knees bent at a right angle. Use only your shoulder to gently place some pressure on your core by moving your elbow closer to the opposite knee. You won't bend far right now, and that's okay. Change between your elbows, and stop if you feel any pain.

With any strengthening exercise, don't pull your muscles too tight. Gradual momentum gets you there. Any exercise in the first six weeks should never make you feel uncomfortable. Avoid intense ab workouts that strain your muscles beyond comfort. Speak to your doctor about ab workouts if you were diagnosed with *diastasis recti* after birth, which is a separation of the abdominal muscles. You should also immediately stop if you see any bulging on your stomach. Your exercise in the first six weeks shouldn't be strenuous. If you find yourself breathless, you've gone too far. You should still be able to have a conversation while exercising. You won't be able to sing, but you'll be able to talk. Any exercise you add should also not place strain on your back. Make sure your back is supported against the floor during workouts.

ELEMENT TWO: DIET

The second element of physical health is nutrition. Everything you eat can impact your mental health. It's not just about losing the baby pounds. It's about giving your body what it needs to keep your mothering journey enjoyable. Nutrition can't miraculously cure PPD or PPA, but it can lay the foundation for your body and mind to feel better postpartum and in the years that follow. Again, better nutrition is an ongoing lifestyle choice that could help you keep your moods aligned. The fact that there are so many unknowns in what causes PPD, research has focused on the hormonal changes our bodies experience after birth.

A systematic review by the University of Colorado Anschutz Medical Campus was published in *Nutrition Research Reviews*, and it shed light on the connection between nutrition and PPD (Ellsworth-Bowers & Corwin, 2012). The researchers focused on what is known as the psychoneuroimmunology connection, which is the link between how we feel, the functions in our brains, and how our immune system functions. Our feelings can create an avalanche of consequences throughout our immune systems and the way our brains function, including our neurological hormones. However, the study of psychoneuroimmunology suggests that the same effects can happen in reverse. Your hormones can impact your physical well-being and vice versa. Part of your physical well-being is nutrition. Everything you eat can impact the way you feel, the hormones flowing in your body, and the way your brain functions.

Consider how hormones also cause "pregnancy brain." They're influenced largely by what you eat. The research at Colorado University examined how specific nutrients, vitamins, and minerals interact with hormones in moms with PPD. The body needs certain nutrients and micronutrients to maintain a healthy immune system and a balanced mental state, and the moms who suffered from PPD appeared to have a deficiency of certain nutrients. Among the nutrients researched, vitamin D seemed to stand out. Lacking certain nutrients can increase your risk of feeling depressed. Reintroducing them can help you keep your hormones and immune system in check. A strong immune system means less pain, stress, and a shorter recovery time. Better hormone regulation also reduces PPD symptoms. Nutrients you should add to your diet include zinc, selenium, iron, folate, omega-3 essential fatty acids, docosahexaenoic acid (DHA), and vitamins D, B-6, and B-12.

These nutrients help you replenish what is already deficient in new moms. Your body needs them to repair tissue and muscles after birth, especially if you had a cesarean. The reason your body naturally becomes deficient is that you've had to supply these nutrients to your growing baby before birth. Breastfeeding moms may also become nutrient deficient if they don't eat right. The deficiency could be worse if you had an eating disorder or you're not eating adequately or qualitatively. The quality of your diet is crucial to combat PPD symptoms. Trying to maintain nutritional quality with a newborn is a challenge, but it's necessary to endure if you plan to overcome depression. You're not trying to perfect your eating habits, but focusing on variety and nutritionally dense foods makes a difference. Your diet should include protein, complex carbohydrates, and healthy, essential fatty acids.

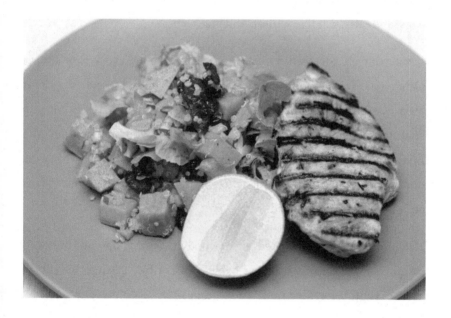

Protein helps your body rebuild tissue and muscle, and it promotes better wound healing while keeping your glucose levels stable. Always look for grass-fed, organic protein, including beef, chicken, seafood, yogurt, eggs, cheese, legumes, seeds, and nuts.

Complex carbohydrates will keep your energy levels up without interfering with your glucose levels, and it aids digestion. Complex carbs are found in whole grains, brown rice, steel-cut oats, quinoa, legumes, fruits, and vegetables without starch. Spinach, cabbage, broccoli, cauliflower, carrots, and other leafy greens are also good options.

Essential fats help your body absorb nutrients. They also regulate hormones and glucose levels while keeping your brain healthy. Some options include extra virgin olive oil, nuts, avocados, seeds, coconuts, eggs, and fatty fish like salmon and mackerel.

Keep yourself balanced by eating a snack or meal every four hours. Otherwise, your blood glucose will fall. Each meal should contain at least one portion of the three options above. Snacks are easy if you stick to fruit and nuts between meals. Adding your nutrients to the mix can be done by taking a supplement recommended by your doctor, or you can find nutrients in natural sources. Some foods contain just what you need.

Calcium needs to be restored as your body takes it from your bones to produce milk and support your baby. You can find calcium in cottage cheese, yogurt, fortified milk, and legumes.

Fatty acids and DHA can promote a better mood and help your baby's brain develop if you're breastfeeding. You can source them in salmon, mackerel, grass-fed beef, organic butter, flaxseeds, and walnuts.

Iron replenishes your concentration and keeps stress at bay. Breastfeeding moms also need more iron. You can find it in poultry, lamb, spinach, beef, and lentils.

Probiotics are another essential as a link was found between the bacteria in our stomachs and the brain, which was published in *Reviews in Neurosciences* (Rios et al., 2017). The flora in your stomach could be affecting your mood. This microbiome is even called the second brain. Maintaining healthy bacteria in your stomach can also fight PPD. Probiotics are found naturally in kimchi, kombucha, yogurt, and kefir.

Vitamin B6, B12, and folate promote better metabolism and breast milk production. They can be found in dark leafy greens, nuts, eggs, whole grains, and red meat.

Vitamin D supports the absorption of calcium. It can be found by getting some sun, but be careful not to burn. Too much vitamin D isn't good. Fortified dairy products, salmon and other fatty fish, egg yolks, and orange juice are also natural sources.

Staying hydrated also aids a balanced nutritional plan to fight PPD and PPA. Water replenishes electrolytes and restores digestive regulation. You may also experience excessive sweating, which is the body's way of shedding extra water retained during pregnancy. This causes dehydration if you're not drinking enough water. You can also add coconut water and herbal teas for hydration, but keep a water bottle close. The rule of thumb is to drink as soon as you feel the slightest hint of thirst.

Invaluable Tips

The thought of focusing on eating healthier with a newborn can be daunting, but some tips make it simpler for you. Planning your meals and preparing them beforehand can save you time and energy. Set aside time weekly to plan your meals for the week, and automate or delegate what you can to make it easier. You can order delivered groceries online or look for a postpartum meal-kit service in your area. You can also cook double to save time in the kitchen by keeping tomorrow's meal in the fridge. Freezing meals ahead of time also helps, and you can bring out a slow cooker for when you're busy with your baby. You'll never stand over a stove all day, so use recipes you can leave in a slow cooker or instant pot. Your meals should be quick to prepare, albeit they must contain complex carbs, protein, and fatty acids.

Asking a friend or loved one to help you with meal preparations can also take a weight off, and you can keep handy and nutritious snacks around the house for those hunger bouts. Boiled eggs, trail mix, yogurt, fresh fruit, and string cheese are good snack options. Speak to your doctor about a quality supplement that contains the nutrients you need. You want supplements that contain methylfolate, which is a bioactive form of folate. Methylcobalamin or adenosylcobalamin are other forms of vitamin B12, and pyridoxal-5-phosphate is vitamin B6. Don't forget your other nutrients. Not all supplements fit well with each mom. That's why you must discuss it with your doctor.

One secret to eating well postpartum is to listen to your intuition. Your body knows what it needs. Trust and respect your body to know when you've had enough and when you need more. You're doing your part by adding a nutritious diet, so allow your body to guide you. Don't weigh or measure your food. You don't want to under nourish your body, either. Stay away from weight loss programs. Your body's recovering, so allow it to naturally restore you, weight, and mind.

If you want to boost your nutritional journey, you can add the top foods that make a difference during postpartum recovery. Full-fat Greek yogurt has protein, and vitamin D. Incorporate various dairy products into your day for nutritional boosts. Lentils and beans also contain loads of fiber, iron, and protein, making them a great staple food for new moms. They're especially important in vegan diets. Organic eggs enriched with DHA can be your go to snack. They provide vitamins B, D, and protein. Wild salmon, sardines, flaxseeds, and walnuts contain DHA and omega-3. They pack a powerful punch against PPD. Whole grains like brown rice, oats, and pasta can give you the energy you crave as a new mom. Change your eating habits, and you'll be experiencing the better side of motherhood. Again, it won't cure PPD or PPA, but it will elevate your mood and energy levels.

ELEMENT THREE: REST

Rest may seem like the holy grail of faraway dreams with a newborn, but it's the third element of physical self-care. A study published in the *Archives of Women's Mental Health* examined how disrupted sleep compares to a baby's temperament during the first three months and which one affects PPD more (Goyal et al., 2009). More than 100 new moms participated in the study, and they were assessed during the third trimester and after birth to determine their PPD scores at each time. The temperaments of the babies were also recorded, and so were the sleeping patterns of each mom before she had her baby. The results showed that a baby's temperament didn't increase PPD symptoms in moms at the three-month check-up, but moms who slept less than four hours between midnight and six in the morning or had less than an hour of daytime sleep significantly climbed the PPD ladder. Quite simply, less sleep equals depression.

Sleep and depression have a bidirectional relationship. You can imagine the two conditions playing tug-of-war. As a therapist, we normally find that the two conditions co-exist. Someone who suffers from depression has trouble sleeping. They often have insomnia, which is the inability to fall asleep, stay asleep, and sleep deep enough to cycle through all the necessary stages. However, people with any form of insomnia tend to become depressed because they struggle to cope with daily responsibilities when they have no energy. In the case of postpartum moms, this loss of sleep further complicates things because our bodies restore themselves when we slumber. Our muscles and tissues strengthen as our immune systems are hard at work while we sleep. Sleep deprivation can also upset serotonin, which leads to depression symptoms.

The positive side of the bidirectional relationship is that we can use proper rest and sleep to reduce depression symptoms. Anxiety disorders also play the same tug-of-war game. You're anxious, so your racing thoughts don't allow your mind to rest so you can fall asleep. On the other hand, a lack of sleep disrupts your ability to concentrate, which may cause you to be more anxious because you can't focus on all the facts surrounding your fears. Take a mom who suffers from postpartum OCD. She also can't imagine her baby remaining safe throughout the night, so she gets up every half an hour to make sure they're breathing. After a few days of no sleep, the mother's fears around her baby's safety only explode because her logical mind is too exhausted to even stop the anxious thoughts. Getting enough sleep postpartum can spare you the symptoms of PPA and PPD.

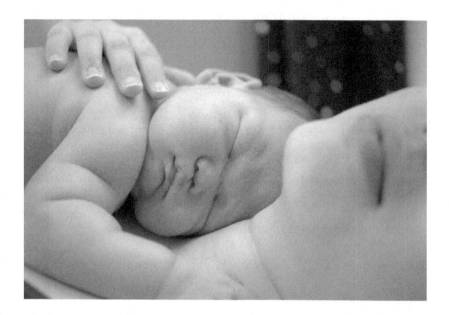

Dos and Don'ts

Knowing that rest can reduce your symptoms is reason enough to make it happen. Many people tell you to sleep when the baby naps, which is good advice, but it's not always possible. Newborns feed on demand, and your symptoms already cause you to lose quality sleep, so half-baked naps don't always work. If you find resting or sleeping opportunities when your baby naps, take them, but some habits should be avoided to improve your sleeping quality and length.

Don't allow yourself to rely on caffeinated drinks, sports drinks, or any stimulating foods that keep you awake. Your goal is to sleep more, not stay awake longer. Avoid all caffeine beverages after two in the afternoon. Chocolate also contains caffeine.

Don't rely on sleeping aids too often, either. Prescription sleeping aids come with warning labels for a reason. You might be too groggy to look after your baby during the night. You may even drop your baby. When it comes to medication for sleep, you can discuss natural melatonin products with your doctor.

Don't ignore the sleep debt you're building. The consequences of sleep deprivation are too vast on your PPD or PPA, whereas getting enough sleep can reduce their severity or symptoms. Watch out for signs of sleep debt, such as difficulties concentrating, blurred vision, sudden appetite changes, moodiness, and forgetfulness.

Don't stimulate your brain with bright lights and noisy electronics before bed. You know you'll be up for your baby frequently, but keep lights dim, noises down, and electronics away when you attend to your baby during the night. Put screens away an hour before you get into bed. The blue light from screens can disrupt your sleep patterns.

Now that you know what shouldn't be done if you want more sleep with a newborn, you can apply some recommended tips to encourage better sleep.

Do go to bed earlier. We tend to think we'll sleep better if we go to bed late, but you're getting up multiple times a night. Try to bring your bedtime one hour earlier for a week, and see if you feel more rested.

Do create a relaxing bedtime routine before you climb into bed. Have a warm bath and ask your partner for a massage to release the tense muscles in your back. Add some lavender oil to your bedroom for a calming effect, and practice a relaxation exercise before trying to fall asleep. Relaxation exercises will be discussed in the next chapter.

Do ask for help from friends, relatives, or your partner when you need rest. Someone can watch your baby while you take a much-deserved nap. Always turn to trusted loved ones to make sure your anxiety doesn't keep you from napping. If you don't have a partner, you can also ask a friend or relative to sleepover for a few nights.

Do share the responsibilities during the night with your partner or trusted friend. Even if you're breastfeeding, you can pump milk during the day and allow your partner to take some night feeds. Work a shared schedule out that allows both of you to bond with and care for the baby, especially in the first few weeks.

Do keep note of your baby's sleeping patterns so you can catch some shuteye while they sleep. Babies will sleep less and less as time passes, and they won't need to feed as much during the night. This takes a few months, though, so keep recording your baby's patterns and introduce them to sleep and feed schedule as early as possible. You can also consider sleep training your baby. It may get harder when you start training them, but the rainbow always comes after the rain. One of the simplest ways you can train a baby from day one is to always put them down before they fall asleep. They must be drowsy, but they must be in their crib before they nod off. This teaches them to self-soothe immediately. Once your baby's down, you can soothe them from a distance by talking or singing to them until they sleep. This way, they don't learn to sleep only in mom or dad's arms.

Do create the best sleep environment for you and your baby, even if they sleep in the nursery. Always keep the room dark, and the thermostat turned to cool. Close the windows to block noise, and purchase a white noise machine to help both of you sleep. Consider whether your bedroom and the nursery look like they welcome sleep. Your bedroom should also only be for intimacy with your partner and sleep, nothing else. This slowly teaches your brain that lying on the bed means it's time to relax.

Do find ways to relax deeply, even when you can't fall asleep. Listen to relaxing music, read a book, or spend a few minutes doing what you love. Any relaxation will help toward replenishing yourself, which you'll learn more about soon.

Even when you do everything right, you may still miss some valuable sleep. Postpartum insomnia is real, and you should commit to getting as much rest as possible. Eating healthier and exercising will also promote better sleep. Combining all three elements lay a foundation for improved physical and mental health.

4

EMOTIONAL SELF-CARE: MINDFULNESS, MEDITATION, AND RELAXATION

You must take care of your emotional well-being while trying to provide the best for your little one. New moms easily forget how to relax, which increases their risk of developing PPD or PPA. However, living in the moment, taking care of your mind, and learning to let things go can improve your emotional well-being. You find your inner calm to manage your symptoms better. Your toolkit against postpartum disorders should include coping strategies to keep your stress levels down. You can't remove stress when you have a beautiful baby, but you can learn how to face it with grit and resilience. The way you respond to the stress of being a new mom and the years to come will determine whether you have a positive or negative experience with parenthood.

EMOTIONAL NOURISHMENT

Looking after your emotional health matters as much as your physical health. What you share with your baby is not just your physical energy. Babies can feel their mom's emotions. Think about it. How does your baby react when you're in a bad mood? Do you feel like they're a greater challenge to soothe? Our emotions tend to rub off on others, including our babies. Being the master of your emotions during the postpartum period can be wonderful for your baby's development. However, the importance of you taking care of your emotions also relates to your ability to cope with motherhood. The symptoms of PPA and PPD can be more profound if you don't know how to respond to fears and obsessive thoughts. You'll feel like you're under the weight of the world if you don't learn how to manage your deep sadness or grief for another life.

You wouldn't be here if you weren't interested in learning how to cope with complicated emotions, so the fact that you're here is already a reason to be proud. The more you prioritize your emotional and physical well-being the same way you care about your baby's well-being, the more balanced you'll be to give your baby the best of you. Ask yourself, do you want to share your best side or the anxious and depressed side? If you want to share the best, you must take care of your emotional health. The more resilient you become, the fewer symptoms you'll experience. You only become resilient by taking care of your emotional needs. Some basic tips can help you nourish your emotional health. Again, prioritize yourself and your baby.

It's fine if the house is a mess and you can't do everything in one day. Permit yourself to skip the housework when you feel drained. You're a new mom, and it takes time to adapt to the juggling act. Another way to ease the emotional implications of being a new mom is to make time for yourself. Ask a trusted friend or your partner to watch your baby while you spend a few moments each day with yourself. Dedicate brief times daily to pamper yourself, whether you love bubble baths, reading, or sipping a cup of tea. Make a weekly habit of self-pampering as well. Maybe you can have a massage while someone watches your baby. If you want to watch an episode of your series, but your mind is distracted by the pile of laundry, urge yourself to let it go. You can always do laundry later or tomorrow. Daily you time is vital to your emotional health, so make it count.

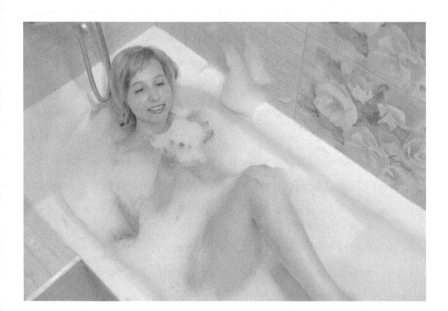

You'll soon realize that the more relaxed you feel, the more time you find to handle the chores anyway. Don't force yourself to do anything that makes you unhappy at this stage. The first weeks after childbirth are a gray area where you can prioritize your energy to improve your mental state to fight PPD and PPA. You can also apply three golden methods to grow resilience—mindfulness, meditation, and active relaxation.

MINDFULNESS

Mindfulness is one of the most valuable skills you'll ever develop. It's the cognitive skill that allows you to experience the present moment fully through your five senses. Additionally, you don't try to change the present or judge yourself. Mindfulness is becoming a regular practice, so two women chose to research the impacts of mindfulness on perinatal depression, which is the onset of depression just before and after childbirth. Professor Sona Dimidjian from the Department of Psychology and Neuroscience at the University of Colorado enlisted the help of professor Sheryl Goodman at Emory University to understand how mindfulness can be used to prevent and treat PPD (Grimes, 2016). They focused on women with a history of depression, knowing they'll be at greater risk before and after childbirth.

The professors took 86 women divided into two groups. One group learned mindfulness while the other group was used as controls receiving conventional treatment alone. These women weren't depressed at the time but had a history. The first group spent eight weeks learning to be present and aware of their current surroundings, the changes to their bodies, and the sensations they experienced through pregnancy and after childbirth. The purpose of this was to see whether PPD could be prevented by adopting mindfulness. The moms who learned mindfulness were 30% less likely to develop PPD within the first year compared to the control moms. Mindfulness can help you prevent symptoms, and it can help you work through existing symptoms of PPD or PPA.

You may already practice mindfulness and meditation, but it seems like it isn't working anymore. That's likely due to a lack of time and not customizing the practice to motherhood. There are many ways you can practice mindfulness as a new mom, and some methods include your baby.

Mindful breathing is one method to use, even with a baby in your arms. Focus your attention on your breath as you gently pull it in through your nose. Take a long breath, and pay attention to how it flows into your abdomen. Hold it for a moment before you allow it gently to flow out of your mouth.

Grounding yourself in a chair while you feed your baby is also mindful practice. Choose a comfortable chair for feeding, and allow your feet to sink into the ground. Notice how your baby's gentle breathing feels against your belly as you notice the temperature of the bottle in your hands or feel the sensations of your baby's feeding on your breast. Pay attention to the way your body folds into the chair, and notice how your feet root themselves into the ground.

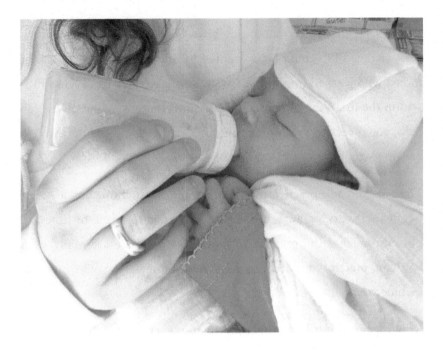

Notice your surroundings if you feel your anxious train of thoughts running away from you. Bring it back to the present by identifying five objects you can see. Say them out loud, and be descriptive about their color, shape, and size. You can also touch the items to help yourself ground in the present.

Practice a body scan when you feel deeply saddened because this is your mind's way of trying to travel to the past. Maybe you're grieving the loss of your body as it was before childbirth. Lie down on a flat and firm surface while you begin your scan on one end of your body. Notice how your toes feel for a moment as they begin to relax slowly. Move to your calves and your thighs, paying attention to each area before moving to another. Keep scanning your body until you reach your mind. Pay special attention to areas that feel uncomfortable. Don't judge these areas. Just allow them to slowly feel better.

Practice daily mindful gratitude by thinking of three things you're happy to experience as a new mom. Maybe your baby made a cute cooing sound this morning. You're happy for the opportunity to be a mom to such a cutie pie. Pay gratitude as mindfully as you can. Notice things you're happy about as they unfold.

Take a mindful walk with your baby. Go to a place that ignites your senses, and feel free to walk over the grass with bare feet. Feel the stroller handlebars between your fingers. Notice how your foot feels as it leaves the ground and connects with it again. Listen to your baby's coos if they're awake. Stand still for a moment, and watch your baby's troller against the backdrop of nature. Pay attention to every sensation you experience on the walk.

Practice a brief mindful meditation when you feel fears creep into your mind. Close your eyes, sit comfortably, and imagine seeing these thoughts and fears as moving objects in your mind. Be silent for a moment while the fears show themselves, and don't try to judge them. Give the fears a physical space in your mind or body as you continue to watch them. You're aware of them in the present moment, but you'll allow them to pass slowly as they lose momentum the more you pay attention to them.

Tune into a sound, such as your baby, with a gentle backdrop of nature or calm, soft music. Focus on your baby's strange noises as you watch them closely. Look into those little eyes while you distinguish their noises from the natural sounds outside the window. Try to imagine what your baby is telling you with those alien sounds.

Practice self-awareness in the present moment when you feel overwhelmed. Just close your eyes and listen to your body, thoughts, and emotions. Be kind and compassionate toward them. Allow them to exist as a part of you, and don't consciously think anything negative toward yourself. Love yourself and allow your emotions to possibly give way to a hint of pride. You're a mom! There's nothing more precious than that. It's okay to feel sad for who you once were. It's okay to feel lost and overwhelmed. Allow your feelings to exist as they are, but imagine what you'd tell your best friend if they felt this way. What kindness could you offer to someone else? Offer the same kindness to your emotions.

Being in the moment with your baby at any time is a way to practice mindfulness. Be aware of every sensory experience while you feed, change, or play with your little one. Give them a massage after bathing them, and allow your hands to ignite the sense of touch. Kiss your little one's tummy while you focus on their funny noises. Watch their tiny little hands cupped into fists. Be close to your baby so that they can see you, too. They can't see far in the first few weeks. Talk to them, and watch those responses, allowing yourself to feel every moment in the present. Think about the softness of your baby's skin while you powder them. This special, mindful time with your baby also helps you bond with them.

Now you have ten simple mindful practices that may even inspire more. Include your baby in your practices, so the two of you can bond, which also eradicates negative feelings and thoughts.

MEDITATION

Meditation has been practiced for millennia. It's not entirely the same as mindfulness, but the techniques can be combined to reduce stress. After all, most of your emotions, fears, and thoughts are being instigated by the stress of a new baby. Harvard Medical School is only one institute that researched the benefits of meditation on stress by looking at the brain (Harvard Health Publishing, 2018). The brain is complicated so that you won't go deep into the details. Two centers in the brain were most intriguing in the research: the medial prefrontal cortex (mPFC) and the amygdala. The mPFC is referred to as the awareness and focus center in the brain, and it's just behind your forehead. The amygdala sits deep in the midbrain, and it's known as the emotional center. Harvard found that both centers are highly active in depressed people, but meditation manages to sever the intense connection between them.

The amygdala is the center that starts your emotional responses. It tells other regions in the brain and body to release stress hormones, which impact the way you function. The mPFC is the part of you that focuses on what you choose to be aware of, so being emotional and being connected to the amygdala can keep you focused on your worries, stresses, and emotions. The research by Harvard proved that disconnecting the two regions responsible for maintaining your stress responses can help you avoid the emotional fallout and focus on happier things. Meditation can successfully fight against PPD and PPA because it changes your brain. However, practice always makes perfect. Meditation requires practice to make the effects last. One session won't always make the world look better. You may need to meditate daily, even if you only manage five minutes.

Meditation also doesn't make your stress or negative thoughts disappear. It helps you understand that your thoughts and emotions may exist, but they don't define you. You don't have to act on them. You can even use meditation to prepare yourself for the day if you feel sad or anxious. It allows you to place a distance between yourself and your thoughts, and you can imagine potential alternatives in your meditation to prepare yourself for the day. You're introducing your brain to a new way of focusing on more than just negative thoughts and feelings. The guided session below will help a new mom who wants to find her inner strength to navigate the day. If this relates to you, feel free to use this guided session every morning before facing the challenges of the day.

A New Morning

Find yourself a comfortable space where you can sit undisturbed for five minutes. Place a blanket or cushion on the floor with a low chair in front of you. Sit cross-legged on this firm and comfortable surface as you allow your arms to rest on the chair gently. Close your eyes and straighten your back as you lean forward and rest your head on your arms. Take a deep breath and allow the air to flow down into your belly where your beautiful baby was recently. This region of your body may feel tender and uneasy. Make sure you're comfortable or sit in a supportive armchair if you're not. You just want to be comfortable as the breath keeps flowing in and out of your body, allowing your abdomen to rise more than your breasts.

Keep breathing gently and deeply as you notice the air flowing down to the core. Allow each breath to bring calmness into this tender area. Pay attention to how the breath flowing out also slowly removes tense feelings from your lower body. Notice if there are any other tender spots in your body, and allow the kind breath coming in to caress the area and relax it more deeply. Feel the air wrap around the areas you focus on, and follow it back through your lungs and out of your mouth as the tension leaves your body. Some thoughts and feelings may come as you're following your breath. It's okay; just let them be. Allow the thoughts and feelings to gently follow the air out of your mind and body as you focus on the deeper relaxation taking over.

Return to your breathing each time a thought steals your attention. Let it go, and allow yourself to relax more deeply. The moment you start feeling calm enough, turn your attention to your imagination. Imagine your day from the moment you end this meditation. Imagine getting up, feeling calm and ready. Imagine going about the things you need to do, but see yourself going about your responsibilities with a new calmness over your mind and heart. See yourself feeding your baby, paying close attention to the calm look on their little faces. Watch yourself putting your little one down for a nap as you continue to calmly face the day. Keep following your routine in your imagination, watching everything unfold in the best way it could.

Imagine yourself feeling relaxed as you attend to your baby. See those heart-warming eyes staring back at you, letting you know that you're doing amazing. Watch yourself take care of your needs as well. Imagine yourself calmly taking the time to make a healthy snack while your baby naps. See yourself not judging any mistakes you *may* make on this beautiful day. You feel no negativity or self-criticism about what you're painting in your mind. You're designing a new day, which may or may not come true. You're so relaxed either way, and you're ready for whatever comes. Your day will be calmer and happier, but you also feel flexible.

See yourself engulfed in a relaxed, trusting state of mind as you continue to progress through this imagined day, and allow your attention to come back to the present moment when you've seen all you need to see. Focus on your breath again, and feel how deeply relaxed you became. Pay attention to the motivation and positive feelings you have about this new day. When you're ready, open your eyes and sit in this calm space for a moment before getting up.

Moving Meditation

Meditation and breathwork aren't all about sitting still. Some forms of meditation help you move your body in a mindful way, such as yoga. We think of yoga as an exercise, which it can be, but it's a combination of moving meditation, mindfulness, breathwork, and exercise. It's also a mental workout and a great way for moms to regain their strength while learning to manage their emotions. A study published in *Complementary Therapies in Clinical Practice* examined how yoga can help for PPD (Buttner et al., 2015). There were 57 postpartum moms divided into two groups, yoga, and waitlist, the latter being used as a control group. All the moms tested high for PPD symptoms. The moms in the yoga group attended 16 classes over eight weeks, and 78% of them showed a dramatic decrease in their symptoms.

The reason postpartum yoga works is that it teaches you to use breathwork while you move your body to encourage healing. This type of moving meditation is called asana. Moving your body while focusing on your breath and the resulting sensations can do wonders for a depressed or anxious mind. The above-mentioned study also found that yoga helped moms reduce their stress hormones. If you're looking to target physical and mental health in one go, yoga is key. Sign up for postpartum classes with a qualified instructor, watch videos for postpartum yoga online, or try these simple poses used for postpartum moms. Yoga is a gentle practice of the mind and body. It shouldn't make you uncomfortable.

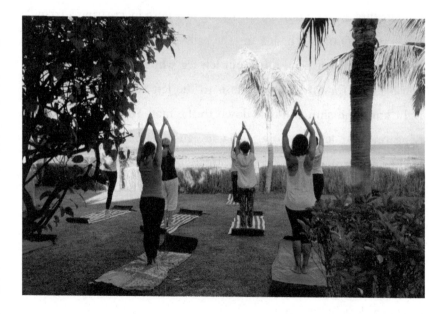

First, there's the extended puppy pose, which helps for relaxation and improved emotional awareness. The Ayurvedic cultures believed this pose opens the heart to see beyond fear and stress. For a simple version at home, place a soft yoga block at the end of a mat if you have them. Sit down gently on your haunches before you lean into the block to rest your elbows on it. Your buttocks should be extended in the air while your hands stay in a praying position. Your head will rest between your arms. Take five slow and steady breaths in and out before gently moving back out of the pose. You'll be able to count more breaths in this pose with practice.

Second, there's the pigeon pose, which works the psoas muscle connected to your stress response. This muscle is tight when you're depressed or anxious, so this pose reduces symptoms. Please do not complete the pose if it hurts. Yoga is about gentle and smooth movements. Enter a downward-facing dog pose by creating a triangle while resting on your hands and the balls of your feet. Rest your head between your arms, and raise your left leg while you inhale. Exhale as you bring it forward and wiggle it to the left side of the mat. Your right knee and shin will ease down to the mat. Your torso should be lying on your left leg now, and you can take a few breaths before leaning forward and reaching for your right ankle with your left hand. Rest your head on your right hand, and allow the floor to support you while you take five to 10 breaths. Release the hold on your ankle, and gently walk your hands forward on the mat. Raise your torso slightly and gently as you start moving your left leg out again. You'll make your way to standing on all fours, and you can move back into a downward-facing dog pose.

Third, there's the warrior pose, which allows you to feel your inner strength again. Stand upright on a firm surface while you interlink your hands behind your buttocks. Spread your legs apart and turn your right leg to face outward. Your left leg and hip must face forward. Bend your left knee to extend past your ankle while you keep your spine straight. Inhale as your arms extend wide open from the back and exhale as they come back to meet each other behind your buttocks. Draw your shoulders back when you exhale, and open your chest while you raise your chin. This is a power pose, so repeat your breathing ten times.

There are many asanas you can learn. Signing up for classes will be the best way you can learn yoga for long-term benefits, and you can take your baby along for some postnatal workouts. It's also a great social experience where you can meet other new moms.

ACTIVE RELAXATION

Active and relaxation don't seem to belong in the same sentence, but you can actively be relaxed. Active relaxation is when you consciously choose to focus on leisure. The more you concentrate on what you're doing in the moment, the more productive your mind becomes. According to psychologist Gretchen Kubacky, slowing down your attention while actively participating in an experience can rewire the brain to learn the actions on a natural level with practice (2013). Actively relaxing means you're consciously choosing and focusing on relaxation. Relaxing is not about doing nothing. If you lie down intending to relax, but you're thinking about everything else, you're not actively relaxing. Here are some ways you can learn to consciously relax daily with a baby.

Finding humor in your experiences can do wonders for your mental health. A longitudinal study published in *Plos One* connected humor and laughter to an improved ability to respond to stress (Zander-Schellenberg et al., 2020). Seeing the funny side of life buffers your mind against stress, anxiety, and depression. Learn to laugh a little. After all, there will be many moments you can laugh at in the coming months and years.

Take a moment to revisit happy memories. Try not to focus on memories that hurt motherhood. Go through an old photo album, or watch the video of the first day your baby came home.

Try drinking some herbal tea because it packs a punch of antioxidants, which is useful in the fight against PPD and PPA. Take a tea break for 10 minutes, and absorb the experience. Smell the tea, taste the warmth on your tongue, and actively participate with all your senses.

Plan your routine around your energy levels. Some moms have bursts of energy in the morning. Others have it in the evening when they want to sleep. Plan one activity during this energy burst where you can enjoy yourself actively. You can also include your baby in this daily ritual. One idea would be to take your nature walks when you feel most energetic. You can also practice a hobby that relaxes you, such as painting, knitting, or scrapbooking. Imagine the great scrapbooks you can show your baby once they grow up?

Give yourself a sweet tooth splurge when you need one. Dark chocolate is a good idea, and it helps your brain release serotonin, elevating your mood naturally. Enjoy your small bar mindfully by noticing how the cocoa engulfs your taste buds.

Start snapping photos because your baby will be moving around before you know it, making it hard to snap a shot. Consciously become one with your camera as you snap images, taking note of the colors, shapes, and other senses you'll remember when you look at the pictures again.

Role-play once in a while to put your day or week in a new perspective. Treat it like a game where you're only allowed to talk about happy moments and positive experiences. Talk to your baby about your week. Let them know about all the wonderful things you saw, heard, and felt. It's good to talk to babies. It helps their communication and social skills.

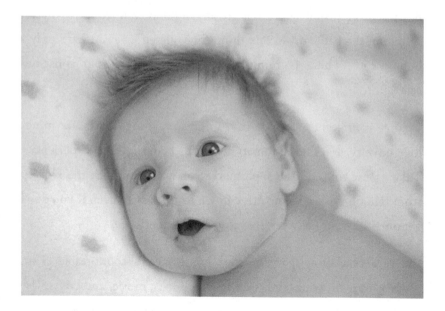

Be playful. A game can always relax us because we're having fun. Board games with your partner or friends can relax you while your baby naps. Play games with your baby as well. Never underestimate what can help their skills develop. Playing peek-a-boo is one of the most recommended games with babies. They love it, and it will get you laughing.

Dedicate one day a week to making meals for the coming week to freeze. Be active in your experience, but avoid this as a relaxation exercise if you don't enjoy cooking. It's not for everyone. If you enjoy it, turn it into a day of fun, laughter, and chats with your baby, who is safely in sight while you chop fresh veggies. Smell the veggies, and taste the spices. Turn it into an active experience with your senses.

Give yourself mommy time each day for at least 10 minutes. During this time, you can read something you enjoy, albeit it should be positive and inspiring. Listen to an audiobook if your partner is watching the baby, or do one thing for yourself, even if that's only a bubble bath. These 10 minutes belong to you and your conscious relaxation.

Change your scenery to give your mind something novel. Our minds love novelty, and they automatically focus better on new experiences. Take a new route to the supermarket or when you pick the kids up from school. Take a scenic drive down to the beach, even if you don't get out with your baby yet. Just absorb the experience.

Create a relaxation space in your home with a comfortable chair. Stock it up with your favorite inspiring books, music, and crafts. Use soothing scents in this corner, such as lavender, chamomile, and vanilla. You can burn scented candles when you spend time in this corner.

Turn responsibilities into fun by singing and dancing while you do the laundry. Your baby will love the show as well. You'll also be laughing. Turn the broom into a mic while you sweep. Any chore or responsibility can be fun if you repurpose them. Feeding your baby can also be a time you conjure up a new story to tell your little one. Maybe the story is from your childhood imagination.

Useful Apps

Turning stress and emotional health around is as simple as actively relaxing. There are also great apps you can download to help you find more ways to relax.

Mood Tools has a digital journal, and it offers video ideas of how to combat stress and other negative emotions. It also comes with a suicide prevention code that will get you to help in your worst conditions if you record certain feelings in the journal.

Peanut is a wonderful app that connects you to other moms in your area. It works similarly to Tinder, except that it's only moms meeting moms based on interests and baby age groups. It helps you get out when you feel overwhelmed.

Happify uses cognitive-behavioral therapy techniques to help you cope with motherhood, and it was developed by psychologists. It gives you ideas of mindful and meditation practices to turn negative moods positive.

Calm is another great app that offers meditations, mindful practices, sleep-inducing sounds, and stretches safe for moms.

Breathe 2 Relax is an app that helps you learn to control your breathing. Using the tools on this app can even help you avoid panic attacks. Hyperventilating is a result of stress, so controlled breathing can naturally help you reduce the effects of stress, preventing a panic attack.

Don't expect yourself to become an emotionally controlled warrior in one day. Practice as many mindful and active relaxation techniques as you can, learn to move in a healing way in yoga, and add meditation to prepare your mind for a new day. Give yourself time, but reach out if you still can't manage your emotions.

5

SOCIAL SUPPORT AND SELF-CARE

A new mom's entire social network changes; sometimes, she becomes too busy to connect with others, and other moms just need to connect with people who understand their journey. Becoming a parent is also challenging for couples, and knowing how to manage your romantic relationship can create a better environment for you, your baby, and your partner. Moms find it even more complicated to maintain and build new relationships when they suffer from PPD or PPA, but our relationships play a huge role in our well-being, so social support is part of your self-care if you want to defeat PPD or PPA. None of us were made to face this world alone, so having social support will be a pivot for you.

A SOCIAL LIFELINE

Being surrounded by loved ones who can support you is a lifeline for moms. It's strange to think you can feel lonely when you just welcomed a baby home, but the isolation is real. New moms can isolate themselves from old friends because they're the first to have a baby. They don't know how to meet new moms, and their romantic relationship feels strained. Both parents being under immense pressure also result in moms feeling lonely. Adding PPD or PPA to the mix, a new mom struggles to flourish in her new role.

A study published in the *Maternal and Child Health Journal* confirms that moms suffer worse from depression if they have no social support (Surkan et al., 2006). Postpartum women at community health centers partook in two surveys. The first one recorded their PPD score, and the second survey measured their social support using the Medical Outcomes Study Social Support Survey (MOS). The results were undeniably in favor of better social support leading to improved well-being. The moms who scored higher on the MOS survey, meaning they had larger support networks, also scored lower on the depression scale. The moms who had two or more close loved ones to support their journeys showed reduced symptoms and risks for PPD.

Social support is also a misunderstood concept. Think about what you need help with versus what your loved ones do when they come over. Your loved ones probably coo over your baby, leaving you to scramble to finish the laundry. When you come back, you feel no better than you did before they arrived. This is one-way incorrect social support can aggravate your symptoms. Even though people think they're helping, and your partner believes they're doing their part if they watch the baby while you cook dinner, in reality, you're not really feeling supported. It's great for loved ones to watch your baby when you want to get things done, but sometimes, you need more. Imagine a friend coming over to do your laundry for you? Imagine your partner hiring a cleaner to make your life easier so you can rest more often? That sounds like better social support.

Even if you think you have a social support network, you may need to rethink how they support you. Speaking to your loved ones helps them understand. You could discuss the possibility of a cleaner with your partner, or you can ask a friend to help make dinner tonight. Postpartum moms who suffer from PPD or PPA feel easily overwhelmed, so looking for ways to ease your load on your terms makes things simpler. Never expect people to know what you need, either. Not only do you need social support, but you must also express your specific needs to loved ones. If you can afford it, hire a midwife who specializes in helping moms with PPD or PPA. Share responsibilities with your partner. Maybe you can take turns at night to feed your little one. This also helps your partner create a secure attachment with the baby if they're fully involved from day one.

Establishing an additional support network with experienced moms can also help fight depression and anxiety. A study published in *The Canadian Journal of Psychiatry* examined the value of speaking to other moms who also suffered from depression (Dennis, 2003). Forty-two moms with high-scoring PPD were divided into a control or a peer support group. The peer support moms received conventional treatment for PPD and benefited from telephonic support from moms who overcame PPD. The control group only received conventional treatment. The peer support group thrived after an eight-week check-up that measured their PPD symptoms again. This study is great for two reasons. First, learning how to cope with PPD from moms who've overcome it works. Second, the peer support was telephonic, which means it also shows how we can still support each other while adhering to social distancing.

The value of postpartum social support is priceless. You may have a close friend or relative with whom you can share your darkest feelings and thoughts. If not, please find ways to develop a support network. Turn to a minister if you're a church-goer. Reach out to local support groups for moms with PPD. Go to your healthcare center, or speak to your doctor or midwife. Don't feel alone or isolate yourself.

MAKING FRIENDS AND SOCIALIZING

New moms should focus on two things. Firstly, you must maintain your relationships with old friends. Secondly, you must make new ones. Making new friends feels awkward at first, but you have the greatest icebreaker. Trying to connect and converse with random new moms is easy because you can talk about your babies. Before you know it, you'll be chatting about chafed nipples and vagina problems in no time. These conversations are awkward for the regular person, but new moms think a lot about the changes to their bodies, and they don't fear talking about it. Making new mom friends is about building a mom tribe to find support, advice, and socialize with women in the same boat as you. Create a tribe by finding baby groups in your local area. Baby cafés and postnatal classes are good places to start.

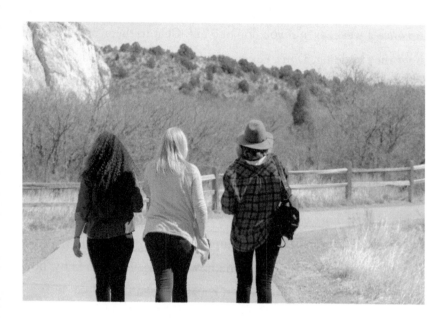

Postnatal classes are also great for professional advice about your recovery after childbirth. Besides, you'll be surprised how every mom is itching to share her most embarrassing and challenging stories, some of which may make you laugh because you can relate. Some postnatal groups also include a counselor. When you arrive, don't be afraid to chat with another new mom. *Postpartum Progress* is a national organization that connects new moms and offers support for PPD by area. For breastfeeding moms who want to make friends, look at an organization called *La Leche League International* (LLLI). Otherwise, visit a local moms club. You can also connect with friends of friends who recently had babies, or you can look at more apps. Apps like *Mush* and *Mom Life* work great for postpartum socializing.

However, the first rule is to maintain your old friendships. Old friends may assume that you've become too busy to make time for them. Communication is the cornerstone of every relationship. Call a friend up once a week, even if you don't go out. Chat to them, and ask them how they're doing. Don't talk about the baby alone, but do let them know if you're feeling blue. Maybe they can come over and help you with something, or you can meet them for a quick juice at a café. Stay connected! You can also set a big date for your first night out after your baby arrives. Let your friends know, so it gives you all something fun to anticipate.

Additionally, don't underestimate your old friends, even if they don't have kids. They might be more supportive than you think. If you're not feeling up to visitors, let them know, but also let them know how much you look forward to seeing them as planned again.

You don't need to pretend to be coping well if you're struggling. Open up to your friends. They might see how much you value your relationship with them. You don't need to cut ties with anyone. Additionally, accept help when a friend offers it. The big day will also come when you have your first night out. Don't plan your first excursion too far away from your baby. Stay local, and allow for two-way conversations with your friends. They probably mind less about your motherhood grumbles than you think, and you'll enjoy listening to stories that don't involve diapers for once. Be the person who invites a friend over as soon as you're strong enough. Try not to make excuses when your friends reach out, either. Motherhood is exhausting, but your social life has to exist to overcome loneliness.

Try to keep promises to your friends, unless something comes up that you can't control.

Maybe you arranged to meet with a friend for coffee, but your relative had an emergency and couldn't watch your baby. This also doesn't mean you have to cancel. Always look for ways to make things work. Take the baby along. You'll feel much better just by spending a few minutes with someone you enjoy. A little secret for those days that seem lonely and all your friends are busy is to reach out to your local community. Neighbor's make great conversations. It might not seem enjoyable when you don't know them at first, but you can randomly talk to neighbors at the local park, over the wall, or even ask the woman down the road if she wants to bring her baby over for a mommy-and-baby visit. Don't be shy because it will only increase your PPD or PPA symptoms. You need a social life, so commit to trying your best with old friends, making new ones, and finding ways to socialize when everyone's busy.

There's only one place you should limit your social life. Social media is not the same as socializing face-to-face. The truth is that it can make PPD and PPA worse if you look at the facts (Green, 2021). Twenty-two percent of parents feel inadequate after looking at boisterous images of babies on Facebook and Instagram, and twenty-three percent feel depressed by the images. Forty percent of parents feel anxious because of parental idealizations on social media. Baby-boasting, exaggerating, mom goals and parenting wins on social media are negatively affecting new mom's moods. We look at these idealistic parenting experiences and wonder why we aren't perfect. We think we're doing things wrong, and our expectations lead to failure. Comparing our journeys to other moms over a platform boasting edited images and selective stories can make us feel like bad moms.

You'll only judge and criticize yourself if you spend too much time on social media. You even lose precious self-care time by being distracted by news feeds, groups, and elaborate stories, which may or *may not* be true. You'll only have an unrealistic picture of motherhood, and you'll succumb to poor parenting advice from people who have no professional background. Social media is not a medical site that offers safe advice. Bad advice can harm your and your baby's well-being. Even worse, you might feel lonelier. Stick to a real social life, and reserve social media and apps for meeting new moms, reading advice from experts, and connecting with friends you know off the platform. Don't be afraid to unfriend or unfollow people, either.

You can also look for support groups on social media run by reliable organizations like the Panda Foundation and Postpartum Progress. Also, only follow positive sources if you must. However, keep in touch with real friends and maintain strong relationships with relatives, especially if you have a sister who doesn't mind hearing about your nipples.

ROMANTIC RELATIONSHIPS

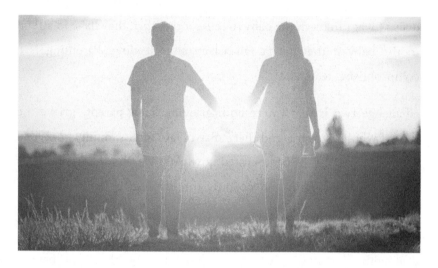

The most important person you want to share a meaningful relationship with is your partner. After all, having a baby connects the two of you for life, so navigating the challenges and maintaining a close connection helps both of you traverse depression and anxiety. There will be challenges in your relationship, but learn to manage them. See what you can both do to improve the dynamics at home.

Challenge one is that different parenting styles cause a stressful clash. Many couples discuss some of what parenting will look like, but parenting styles can erupt if you're both up for a fourth night with a crying baby. Dad believes in soothing the baby, but mom wants the baby to self-soothe after feeding. You and your partner will disagree about parenting styles when you're both exhausted. The solution is for both of you to research your opinions or discuss them with an expert *together*. You both may change your mind about something new. If you can't agree, you can always work on the natural consequence system. Each parent continues with their style, but they have to deal with the consequences if it doesn't work. If your partner doesn't want to teach the baby to self-soothe, then they have to attend to the baby if they won't fall asleep after feeding. Parenting is a compromising team effort.

Challenge two is that you're both grieving. New parents grieve the loss of who they were, and that's okay. Date nights, dinners out, and weekend trips will be complicated now. Allow each other the time to grieve your old selves and do little things to make each other feel special. If you want your partner to transition into their new role, show gratitude for their actions and sentiments. Find new ways to deal with your new roles. Have a no-chores weekend, or have a conversation about anything not related to the baby while the baby naps.

Challenge three is that communications break down, and it's due to both of you being exhausted. PPD and PPA cause a break in communication. Relationships require communication. You have to find moments to listen to each other. You must share your experiences and laugh together.

Moreover, your communication must be positive toward each other. Never blame your partner for anything. Instead of saying, "You never help me!" Rather say, "I'd love it if you could help me with this." You're not accusing your partner of anything, and you're using the invaluable 'I' statement to share your feelings about what their help would mean to you. You can also lead with better communication by acknowledging their feelings first. For example, "I know you're tired now, but I'd love your help with this." Both of you must express yourselves and listen to each other's emotions without adding negative tones or words. Moreover, make time to chat daily.

Challenge four is that both of you may experience PPD or PPA. This is like a candle burning both ends. Both of you must remember that your self-care is essential. Keep yourselves healthy, and allow your partner to take over if you feel overwhelmed. Give each other space to deal with your emotions in self-care rituals, but don't stop talking to each other. The two of you must support each other, or this journey will become a lot harder. And if either of you feels the need to take a break, do it. Couples also need to realize that sometimes, one parent may need to recoup. They might have to take charge of the baby, household chores, and other responsibilities until their partner improves. If you're the one in charge, be sure to keep maintaining your health by eating well, sleeping, exercising, and seeking social support.

Challenge five is that mutual exhaustion leads to conflict. Sleep is a valuable asset to both of you and ensuring you equally get as much as possible will keep your relationship intact. Some moms fear asking their partners for help because they think their partner expects them to be happy and capable. You must ask for help, and playing the divide and conquer game keeps you both healthier. Sure, one partner may work full time, but that doesn't mean the home partner must handle all the responsibilities, especially not at night. Ask your partner if they can handle the last feeding before bed and maybe one during the night. You can also alternate between waking up on different nights. Research by the National Health Institute also found evidence that men's brains don't respond as well to a baby's cries (2015). A woman's brain biologically becomes more attentive to a baby's cries, so don't be too hard on your partner for snoozing when the baby cries at night. Gently wake him up if it's his turn.

Challenge six is that both of you can struggle to find time for yourselves. This can only be solved by working together, planning times daily where both parents have some downtime, even if it's only 10 minutes. Planning ahead automatically reduces any tension between you.

Challenge seven is that "couple time" becomes "family time." Two people cannot remain intimately bonded if they don't have time alone together. Family time isn't the same thing. Firstly, you must dedicate time together, whether you're going for dinner, discussing plans for the future, or just giving each other a back rub. You can both choose a time daily where you can be emotionally intimate with each other. Maybe you can have this special time just after the last feeding before you go to bed. It may be interrupted by your baby, but this gives you daily time for each other. You can also get a trusted relative to watch the baby when you go for walks, dinner, or anywhere for an hour together. Neither of you should feel guilty about these times away from your baby. The better your collective mental health becomes, the better parents you become.

Challenge eight is that sex becomes a myth after a baby arrives. Couples need intimacy, but there's a little secret here. Intimacy doesn't only mean sex. Emotional and physical intimacy can be achieved with meaningful conversations, sharing your passions, and giving each other a bedtime massage. And when the time comes, sex can slowly return, even if you're exhausted as a new mom. Realize that it won't be the same at first. Your doctor may give you the green light, but it can also still be uncomfortable. Make sure both of you are ready, so prepare to rest before sex, and get each other properly aroused. Sex may not be very appealing for new moms after all the changes, but it's crucial to restore your intimacy with your partner.

Romantic relationships need sex, and if a new mom really wants to keep things happy while she's still recovering, there's nothing like a "little handy sacrifice." Intercourse, foreplay, and little naughty moments can help both of you blow off steam, and it shows your partner how much you still want them. You can also get in the mood by planning sex, even if this doesn't seem sexy. It gives you both time to build your passion and desire before making love. It can also help you prevent being disturbed by the baby if you have someone trusted caring for them. Know that it's okay to feel tired while you both remember why you love each other. Plan and prepare around better rest for both of you to enjoy the experience.

Challenge nine is that financial worries can creep in. You may also be at home longer than expected if you're suffering from PPD or PPA. Teamwork is recommended here. Discuss the future of your finances with each other, and choose to support each other's decisions. Your partner may not be able to carry you on their salary alone, so you'll have to prepare to return to work. You might decide to make some budget cuts. Working as a team is the only way both of you can know what to prepare for and expect. Not talking about financial fears can cause stress and relationship failure.

Challenge ten is that your in-laws may spend a lot of time at your home. Sure, it's great to have your mother-in-law helping with the baby, but no one likes being told what to do, how to handle the baby, and how to be a mother. The way around this is to let your partner know how you feel. Communicate openly with them without using negative language. You can suggest that your in-laws come around once a week, and you'll make sure you're ready for them.

Challenge eleven is that forgiveness can be a hard pill to swallow. Your emotions as a new mom can be all over the place, so be sure that they don't impact your judgment. Your partner is also tired and makes mistakes as a new parent, so be open to forgiving them. Both of you must forgive mistakes and move on.

Challenge twelve involves the disagreements that lead to conflict. How do you solve it? There are ways to manage conflict better. Ask for specific changes or help, and never accuse or direct blame at your partner. Always apologize for hurtful words and accusations, and only use positive communication to share your feelings and validate theirs. You can ask your partner how they feel, or you can paraphrase what they said to validate their feelings. When you mention how you feel, don't use the word 'you' if you can help it. Don't say, "You make me mad." Say, "I feel mad." Limit your responses to allow your partner to speak. Listen attentively to what they say before you respond with positive words again. Take a 20-minute break from each other if you need to cool down. Don't leave without saying you'll be back in 20 minutes. Don't bring the past up, either. Always only discuss what is necessary now. Finally, make contact with your partner. Touch your partner's hand and look them in the eyes. This allows you to stay connected.

Other than addressing the common problems that arise between partners after a baby comes, you should also commit to making time for each other. Both of you should work on keeping your relationship strong while you're finding your feet in your new roles.

As a new mom, you have what it takes to make your social life a priority now. It's part of your self-care. You'll feel a lot worse if you have PPD or PPA and feel alone.

6

YOUR SPECIAL RELATIONSHIP: BONDING WITH YOUR BABY

One of the most precious relationships in life is that between a mother and a child. PPA and PPD may prevent you from bonding with your baby the way you want to. Just like any other relationship, this one has a double-sided advantage. When moms create a secure attachment with their babies, their symptoms can alleviate because they start experiencing the positive side of motherhood. Some hormones are connected to bonding, and they can help you reduce negative symptoms.

On the other hand, having a secure attachment with your little one will give them a better start in life. The first relationship they build is either with their mom or dad. It sets the stage for every relationship in their lives. If you want to reduce your PPD and PPA while giving your baby the best start you can, you should bond with them.

SECURE ATTACHMENTS

A secure attachment is one where you emotionally interconnect with your baby, and it allows them to develop their skills, communicate healthily with others, and create healthy relationships, even in adulthood. They grow into confident children who enjoy being with other people, and they have no problems sharing their feelings or seeking support when they need it. Moreover, a child with emotional regulation can also bounce back from failures and overcome losses later in life. The way moms bond with their babies is that they respond to their baby's needs, including emotional cues like crying. This allows a child to feel safe and develop emotional regulation, which even improves their cognitive skills. Your baby will also learn to trust you and communicate their needs better, which is something that could make so much difference when they get older. We learn empathy, compassion, love, and being able to connect with other people in infancy. When two people connect, a hormone called oxytocin is released, which makes both persons feel secure and loved. It's known as the bonding hormone.

You're biologically designed to fall in love with your baby if you can just compassionately move yourself past anxiety and depression symptoms. PPD and PPA can prevent a secure bond, even though the bonding hormone may relieve the negative symptoms from postpartum conditions. According to Princeton University's review of relationships and behavioral aspects in early childhood, a survey of 14,000 children in American showed that 40% of them lacked secure attachments (Huber, 2014). These children are more likely to have behavioral and educational challenges without secure attachments.

The release of the love hormone during close contact and emotional bonding with your baby also benefits both of you. Not only does it promote better learning and development for a baby, but it also reduces the negative hormones playing ping pong in your body. You feel more caring, loving, happy, empathetic, and sensitive to the needs of others, which helps you start responding better to your baby.

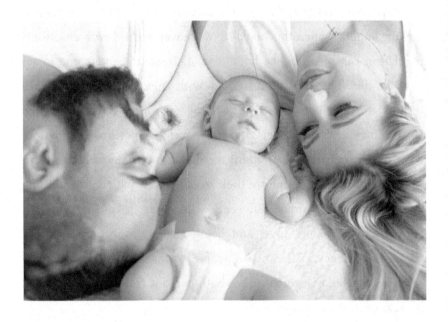

You can also fight the fatigue that comes from lost sleep when you bond deeper and realize how much you love this little person. The endorphins released boosts your energy and motivates you. Creating a secure attachment when you suffer from PPD or PPA can be challenging, but it's worth the effort for both of you. Sometimes, all it takes is making skin-to-skin contact with your little one. Watch for signs that you're not bonding with your baby. You may feel like they're a total stranger, or they don't seem to know you well. Your feelings toward your baby are mixed and confusing, or your baby may show negative feelings toward you. Maybe they cry when you hold them, but they don't cry when someone else does. You may also feel like you lack the energy to care for them, and no matter how hard you try, you can't seem to get the response you want from them. These are signs that your PPD or PPA are interfering with your bonding process.

Don't fear failure in establishing a secure attachment with your baby. That will only elevate your anxiety. Know that you can start developing a secure bond, and things will change, even if you have a baby who doesn't behave positively toward you. It's never too late to deepen your connection. But first, you should know what a secure attachment is. An attachment is an emotional connection babies share with all their caregivers, but a secure attachment is the kind that allows a baby to flourish in their social and emotional development. It's the kind where your baby senses your dependability, and that grows as you attend to their needs and emotional cues in as much a consistent way as possible. Don't fall victim to the myths about secure attachment, either.

Myth one is that secure attachments are natural because you birthed your baby. Babies have unique nervous systems that are still developing, and their needs may not be the same as yours. Just because you're the mom doesn't mean your baby will respond positively to the same things you enjoy.

Myth two is that moms think they lack a secure attachment because they don't know their baby's cues and needs. Don't expect yourself to understand a baby's needs when they aren't even sure what they need yet. Mistakes will be made, and the best thing a mom can do is repair the temporarily lost connection. Remember that attachment is a two-way street as well, just because you don't know their needs. Your baby also needs to read your cues, and a temporary failure to do so doesn't mean you're not securely attached.

Myth three is that love and secure attachment are the same things. Bonding isn't always natural for moms, even if they love their babies. Building a secure attachment is about addressing your baby's needs, trying to make sense of their emotions to soothe them, and reducing your stress around them.

Myth four is that babies can be spoiled if all their needs are met. Bonding and teaching your baby emotional regulation and social skills do the opposite of spoiling them. They learn to trust others, and they become independent because they can manage their emotions.

Myth five is that babies can bond securely with multiple caregivers. Babies will form many close relationships and attachments with their caregivers, but they're likely to only form one secure attachment, which will be to their primary caregiver, being you or your partner.

Secure attachments are a process that requires dynamic and mutual interactions between you and your baby. It's an exchange of non-verbal communication with a newborn and the coming months. Your baby will listen to your tone of voice, watch your gestures and facial expressions, and feel your emotions. In return, your baby will cry, coo, babble, or mimic your facial expressions to communicate with you. Eventually, they start smiling, pointing, and saying their first words. Your baby knows you're communicating with them, and they use this unspoken way of communicating their needs back to you. Neither of you can understand each other yet. A secure attachment will flourish if your initial non-verbal interactions are successful, even if only most of them succeed. Expressing your PPD or PPA symptoms in your interactions with your baby will put them in a bad mood because they feel your emotions. Sharing consistently positive interactions can increase your chances of a secure attachment.

It may be challenging to form a secure connection if your baby had problems in the womb or during delivery, was sick right after delivery, or has a compromised nervous system. Babies born prematurely, left with multiple caregivers every day, or separated from their parents at birth can also struggle to connect. Parents can battle if they suffer from PPA, PPD, alcohol, or drug problems. High stress levels, living in an unsafe environment, or having negative or abusive memories from your childhood can also prevent bonding. Recognize your challenges, and work toward establishing the best bond you can with your baby from now.

BONDING BASICS

Knowing the basic secrets behind secure attachments can help you move through the challenges or symptoms of PPD and PPA.

The first secret is that secure bonding doesn't mean you must be with your baby every minute of every day.

The second secret is that mistakes are expected and a part of this journey. Never judge yourself or think you must be perfect. Maybe you take longer to bond than a friend. Any mistakes you make when addressing your baby's needs must also be acknowledged. Show your baby how you're trying to improve each day. Try to become more consistent in your interactions.

The third secret is to be prepared for disappointment. Some moms will push their babies away for fear of not developing a secure attachment. Just remember that you're not perfect, and neither is your baby. Trying your best at all times is the greatest way you can attend to their needs. If you feel emotional, step back and allow someone else to take over.

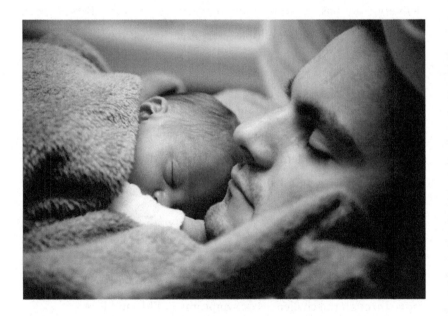

The fourth secret is that dads should also attempt to create a secure attachment with their babies. It may be more challenging, but it will also come in handy if a mom is feeling too low to interact positively with her baby. Dads can sing to their babies, change them, bathe them, feed them, and have conversations using their body language and facial expressions. They can play games with a baby like peek-a-boo. Dads should hold their babies as much as possible to create a healthy attachment.

The fifth secret is not to take your baby's responses personally. Don't feel like you've done something wrong if they turn away from you. Give them a moment to explore what their little eyes are trying to focus on and continue being the consistent mom they need. Babies can go through phases where they appear to be interested in everything but mom or dad. It's natural, so don't be alarmed.

The sixth secret is to get to know your baby. You won't know them well at first, but they also don't know you. You want to learn their cues, even if you get a few wrongs at first. Pay attention to your baby's facial expression and body movements while they make sounds. Familiarize yourself with the different sounds and what your baby's mood might be. Moms quickly learn the hunger cry, but what about that cry to see a smile from mom? More importantly, notice what makes your baby happy. Try different voices, facial expressions, and even touching them in certain ways. Some babies love being massaged, and others can be fussy. It's a matter of trial and error.

The seventh secret is that you won't always respond immediately to your baby's needs. Babies just need to know they're recognized, and they must trust that you'll address them soonest. Being as consistent as possible teaches your baby that mommy will help soon.

Once you have the basics, there are many ways you can bond with your little one. Skin-to-skin contact is highly recommended. That's why the nurse probably brought your little one to you as soon as they were born. Touching someone's skin helps us release the love hormone. Hold your baby close while you sing to them, give them a massage for those developing little muscles, and blow kisses on their tummies. The benefits of skin-to-skin contact were published in *Nursing for Women's Health* (Moran-Peters et al., 2014). Both of you will sleep better and experience less stress. Your baby will gain weight easier and have improved brain development. If you're still at the hospital, you may even be discharged earlier. Nurses encourage skin-to-skin contact in the first 30 minutes after birth, but moms who had a cesarean can also benefit by bonding as soon as possible. Baby massages are a great way to have skin-to-skin contact, and you can watch guided videos online to give your baby a full rub down.

Communicating with your baby is another bonding experience. Sure, they can't understand your words yet, but they love seeing your smile, hearing your laughter, and watching the funny faces you make for them. Always remember that communication at this stage is non-verbal, but singing and reading to them also helps to develop their language skills to find their first words in a few months. Some moms even teach their babies simple sign language before they talk because this helps them communicate their needs when you can't understand their babbles. Start using hand gestures when you speak to them, and you can talk about anything as long as you keep a happy and loving tone of voice. Allow them to respond with those little coos and babbles by taking breaks between what you're telling them, and encourage them to smile back at you.

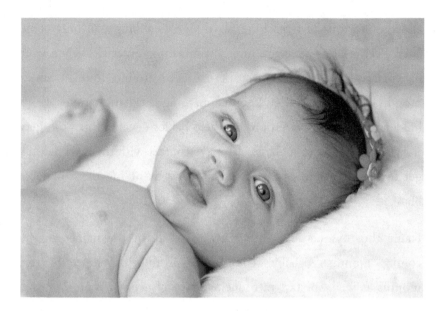

It's also never too early to sing them lullabies and read them age-appropriate stories from board books they can feel. Babies need to develop their fine motor skills, and you can do this by allowing them to feel the texture of baby books. Hold them close while you read a story, and sing in a positive and happy tone. Anything that stimulates their senses helps them develop various vital skills, but it can also improve your bonding because they want to learn about this new world with their senses. That's why babies put everything in their mouths when they start crawling. They can learn more about you if they feel, see, and hear you.

Play with your baby, which also allows bonding and development to co-occur. Use black and white images with newborns because they don't see colors yet. They also love seeing faces but know they can only see about 10 inches away for the first few weeks. Always hold your face near if you're playing with them. Their focus will increase, and they'll soon start reaching for things. Grabbing will only come later. Peek-a-boo games are highly stimulating, especially when your baby starts developing object permanence around four to seven months. This means they know something's still there, even if it's hidden. Peek-a-boo variations can help babies develop this skill. Play the classic version to make loads of eye contact with them while they get to see your smile, or you can use toys by hiding them under a blanket.

Name the toys because your baby might learn the names in the coming months. A baby's color vision is fully developed by five months as well, so start introducing colorful toys with noisy music. Sensory play is vital for a baby to develop all their skills. A rattle can even help them to start tracking moving objects. Give them plenty of playtime with educational baby toys, and be involved. Stick close to them, and make as much skin-to-skin contact as possible. Introduce them to various textures as well. You can even play a game of fabrics by gently moving different textures over their little tummies and faces to make them smile.

Look for any reason to bond with your little one, and encourage your partner to do the same. It will help you on those down days when you need someone else to watch the baby.

BREASTFEEDING TO BOND: YES OR NO?

There's a classic debate about whether moms who breastfeed can bond easier with their babies. A study published in the *International Journal of Psychiatry in Medicine* confirms that breastfeeding may even reduce the risk and symptoms of PPD for up to four months after childbirth (Hamdan & Tamim, 2012). Breastfeeding has long been known to effectively help moms bond with their babies, but it's also not the only way. There are still cases of women developing PPD symptoms while breastfeeding, albeit it's less common. The condition is called Dysmorphic Milk Ejection Reflex, which is a sudden onset of depression symptoms while you're breastfeeding. One factor that may determine whether breastfeeding will reduce symptoms of PPD and increase the likelihood of a secure attachment for you depends on *what you want.*

Do you want to breastfeed or bottle-feed your baby with formula? If you want to breastfeed your baby, the motivation and excitement alone can increase your chances of bonding this way. If you're not into the idea of breastfeeding, or you can't for reasons you know, you'll find ways to bond with your baby without a nipple between you. There's no right or wrong answer here. It depends on what you want and what makes you feel comfortable. It's also perfectly normal if you can't breastfeed your baby. Some moms struggle with breastfeeding, so *never* feel guilty about your choices. You're the mom, and as long as you're prioritizing you and your baby's well-being or attachment, you have no worries. Always choose what feels right for you and your bundle of joy. If you choose formula, there are many ways you can still bond with your baby. You can still use skin-to-skin contact. Lay naked with your baby, but keep a cover over both of you if it's cold.

Bottle feeding also doesn't mean you can't communicate with your little one. Have baby talk sessions while you lie naked together. Allow your baby to cuddle close to you and sing them lullabies. Use your hand gestures and facial expressions when you read them stories, and play games to stimulate their senses. Comfort your baby with a gentle voice every day, even if they don't need you at the time. Stare into their little eyes while you keep your face close enough to communicate with them. Any of the bonding exercises already mentioned can work for a mom who uses formula. The only thing you'll be skipping is the breastfeeding part. If you want to lie naked next to your baby, and they show interest in your breasts, but you can't breastfeed them, wear a sports bra while you still make contact with them. You can also just hold them in your arms without wearing a shirt.

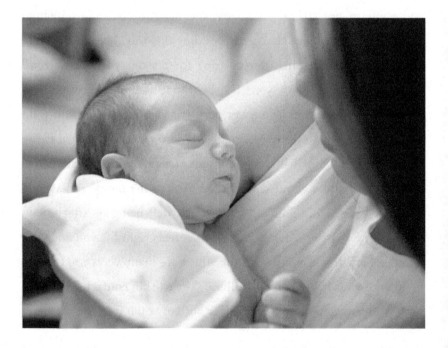

The most important thing to remember when bonding with your baby is that you're not perfect, they're not perfect, and you can both be imperfect together. A secure attachment must also be an ongoing effort, even when your baby turns into a toddler. You can do this, no matter how you feel right now. It doesn't matter how your bond looks at the moment; you can still achieve a close, healthy, and secure relationship with your precious baby.

7

WHEN YOU NEED SOMETHING MORE: TREATMENT AND MEDICATION OPTIONS

Self-care is an empowering way to prevent and manage PPD and PPA, but sometimes, you need more than just meditation and a good chat with your partner. You still need self-care to build the foundation of where you want to go with your mothering journey, but it's also okay if you need additional healthcare services. Admitting that you need help will be your greatest sign of bravery. Knowing when to seek help, how to discuss your options with your doctor, and what treatment options are available can place you in the driver's seat to be the mom you deeply desire.

CHOOSING HELP

Physical, emotional, and social self-care will be the cornerstones of your improved mental health if you suffer from PPD or PPA, but reaching out for professional help, in some cases, will enhance your road to recovery so you can enjoy your gorgeous baby. If you're someone who's worried about a loved one suffering from PPD or PPA symptoms, and it doesn't seem like they're coping, please consider reaching out for help on their behalf. You can make them aware you want to help, but be their support system which finds resources, options, treatment plans, and just someone who stands by their sides. People don't always know they're suffering from depression or anxiety. It makes a huge difference if a loved one can compassionately help them become aware of it. Compassion is the only way to make your guided help work. If you suspect your loved one is showing signs of postpartum psychosis, please get them to help immediately.

For a new mom who recognizes how much you need and want help, a time may come when you need to reach out to a professional. Don't allow embarrassment to make you reluctant. You won't always see your symptoms worsening, or if they're already bad, so it helps to discuss your symptoms with a doctor as soon as you realize there's a problem. The longer you wait, the longer your return to a better way of feeling will be. Watch out for signs that your baby blues have turned into something more. Consider whether they've existed for more than two weeks, seem to be getting worse, or you're finding daily tasks challenging. Call a doctor to schedule an appointment if you find it difficult to care for your baby, or you're thinking of harming yourself or the baby.

The same applies to PPA. If you feel excessive worry, dread, or you can't stop thinking about the worst-case scenario, please seek help. Feeling overwhelmed, panicky, or like you have no control are also reasons to seek treatment. Ask for help if you experience any symptoms you've learned about in this book, and they're not clearing after two weeks, including postpartum OCD, panic disorders, and depression. Immediate help is recommended if you have signs of postpartum psychosis, suicide, or thoughts of harming your little one, and you don't feel bad about them. Again, the National Suicide Hotline is **1-800-273-8255**, but you can also call a loved one, religious leader, or your primary physician. You can also reach out to an obstetrician-gynecologist, your baby's pediatrician, or a midwife. When you choose to reach out to a professional, use these tips to help you speak to them about your condition.

Firstly, choose someone who makes you feel comfortable, irrespective of the type of doctor. Maybe you have a good rapport with your primary physician. Choose someone who won't dismiss your feelings and concerns. You want a compassionate person, and you can even ask them to refer you to someone who deals with postpartum disorders.

Secondly, don't be hesitant to speak to your doctor about the scariest and most personal feelings. They must understand what you're experiencing. Talk about your symptoms in detail. Your symptoms don't define you as a mother. They merely show a temporary lapse in your mental health. Don't allow your fears of what others will think to deter you from receiving the treatment that will promote your mental health, either. Even if someone calls you a bad mother, walk away from their ignorance, and do what you need to right now. Taking medication doesn't make you a bad mother, either. In fact, your motivation to improve yourself for your baby makes you a better mother than the critics. Besides, you shouldn't surround yourself with people who enlarge your fears about mental health treatments just to hide their insecurities. This journey feels so much better when you're surrounded by positive people.

Thirdly, be prepared when you arrive at your appointment. If you're suffering from PPA or PPD, chances are you'll forget things easily. Make notes, research your conditions, write down your symptoms and experiences, and take the information to your appointment. The more you can share with a doctor, the better chance you have of receiving the right treatment. A doctor who doesn't dismiss your concerns will at least screen you for PPA and PPD. You should also request that your doctor does a thyroid test and blood count to rule out any other reasons for your symptoms. You know what may cause these conditions now, so ask them to check it so you can know you're not depressed for physical deficiencies.

Fourthly, ask all the questions you have when your doctor suggests a treatment, especially medication. Ask them how it would affect breastfeeding. Always let your doctor know you're breastfeeding. Many of the medications recommended today will not affect the secretion of milk or pass effects along to a baby, but your doctor doesn't know you're breastfeeding unless you mention it. Don't think of any question you may have as silly. If you're on medication, ask for a follow-up appointment so you can let the doctor know whether it's working well for you. Many primary physicians can handle medication treatments, but you can also ask for a referral to a mental healthcare professional if you want therapy options. They can also treat you with medication while offering therapy treatments.

Finally, know you're in the wrong place if your feelings are being dismissed as regular new mom nervousness or the baby blues. Some doctors aren't as compassionate as we need during our postpartum journey. It's okay to ask for a referral or just find another doctor. You have a right to be part of your mental health treatment plans and options. You should also make it clear to your doctor that you'd like to be part of the decisions and know more about the options. It's also your right to feel supported and informed. It's a good idea to take your partner or another loved one with you so you can have a second opinion. Your doctor may also be quite thorough, offering you various options. You may not remember them all, and your partner can be your second memory. This also adds social support to seeking help for your mental health.

Don't allow your mental health to be managed by someone else alone. Professionals might take over if you're experiencing psychosis, but that's okay. Trust them to help you feel better. However, in mild or moderate PPA and PPD, you can have just as much choice in your treatment plans as your doctor. You can say no to one treatment and ask for more information about others.

TREATMENT OPTIONS

On the brighter side, there are many different treatment options to consider. From individual therapy to group sessions, and from medication to hormone therapy, you'll find an option that feels right. Being guided by professionals who specialize in postpartum conditions combined with a compassionate and understanding nature can already make you see a silver lining. Some doctors may recommend   psychotherapy   combined   with   medication. Psychotherapy is also known as talk therapy. You'll be able to share your thoughts and feelings, and you'll learn how to respond better to stressful situations. The most common medication prescribed during the postpartum period is called a selective serotonin reuptake inhibitor (SSRI). According to Ohio State University, some SSRIs like Citalopram can even renew connections in a part of the brain damaged by stress during pregnancy (2014). Know your options, and you'll feel more confident about your recovery.

Psychotherapy

Psychotherapy is also not a one shoe fits all kind of treatment. There are various options to consider, depending on your symptoms and the recommendations from your doctor.

Cognitive-behavioral therapy (CBT) is a popular choice for moms with postpartum OCD and PPA. CBT therapists understand that our thoughts can change the way we feel and behave, so this type of therapy helps you recognize your underlying thoughts before you work toward changing them. You'll also learn how to distinguish a realistic thought from an unrealistic one, and you'll identify your automatic thoughts, which are created by beliefs. CBT is a two-person therapy, which means you're fully involved and in control. The therapist may also show you coping strategies you can practice daily, and they can give you homework to surface those distorted beliefs that cause your unrealistic thoughts. There's also a mindfulness-based CBT, known as MCBT.

Couples therapy is a great option if you and your partner are struggling to communicate, return to intimacy, or experience negative interactions that cause constant distress. The therapist focuses on the most important part of relationship healing, which is communication. They'll teach you both how to communicate and listen to each other effectively, and they'll help you find ways to compromise with goals and parenting styles.

Dialectical behavioral therapy (DBT) may be a combination of group and individual therapy, which also works similarly to CBT. The purpose of DBT is to teach you how to cope with unruly thoughts, regulate your emotions, tolerate distress, and become mindful. You'll also gain better interpersonal skills, which helps you bond with your baby and loved ones during this stressful time.

Eye movement desensitization and reprocessing (EMDR) therapy is commonly used to treat moms with postpartum post-traumatic stress disorder (PTSD). A specialized therapist will use specific desensitization techniques to help you reduce your responses to a traumatic experience. One method used in EMDR is bilateral stimulation. You'll be guided into a visualization while your left or right side of the brain is stimulated with bilateral sounds, eye movements, and tactile stimulation. This helps you reprocess the memory more effectively. EMDR is not only used to reprocess traumatic memories. It can also help new moms effectively process positive memories about their experiences.

Group therapy can work for PPA and PPD. A psychotherapist will use the power of community support to help new moms learn about their conditions and find their reasons for interpersonal distress. You'll be surrounded by new moms who also have challenges daily, and you'll learn as a group to use lifestyle changes and stress reduction techniques while you make some new friends.

Interpersonal psychotherapy (IPT) is an effective treatment for PPD. It's a short-term therapy that lasts between 12 and 16 weeks, but it targets the symptoms of PPD, helping you find ways to reduce them. Your therapist will be direct with you, but they'll give you insight into your depression symptoms and alternative ways of feeling. The four skills you'll learn in IPT are role transition, grief management, interpersonal disputes, and interpersonal deficits. Learning to manage grief will help you overcome the life you grieve from before motherhood, and role transitioning will help you accept and be comfortable with your new role. You'll learn how to deal with the loss of independence and cope with the changes in your relationships, family dynamics, and sense of self. Interpersonal disputes are the expectations you had of this journey and intimacy after childbirth, and the therapist will help you realize your unmet expectations. Interpersonal deficits are when people struggle to build healthy attachments, even in other relationships. You'll be shown how to improve your attachments.

Psychodynamic psychotherapy is what you likely expect when looking for talk therapy. Your thoughts and beliefs are influenced heavily by your past experiences so that they might ask you about childhood memories, your relationship with your parents, and the dynamics of your childhood home. This form of therapy works to unravel the source of your beliefs. For example, you think you're a terrible mom, which prevents you from seeing the great things you provide your baby. You might surface a belief that started when you were a child. Maybe your parents always doubted themselves, which didn't allow for a secure attachment, but you remember how many great things they did for you. Psychodynamic psychotherapy is about finding the 'ah' moments. Sometimes, awareness of the false beliefs we hold is enough.

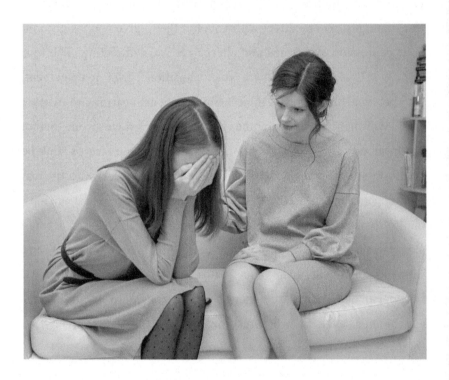

Solution-focused brief psychotherapy doesn't focus on past experiences but rather on the specific problems a mom faces right now. The therapist will also focus on your strengths and skills to help you solve the issues you're experiencing. The purpose of this therapy is to set goals and find solutions. This is also a short-term therapy that only lasts a few sessions.

Only you can decide what therapy types sound best for you. Doctors will recommend options, or you can ask a therapist which type they use before proceeding, but it's your choice. Different moms respond differently to various treatment options.

Medication

Medication might be recommended to treat PPA or PPD. One of four options may be discussed.

Atypical antidepressants are a newer form of antidepressants used to target neurotransmitters in your brain, and they work faster than the older ones. This is an option for PPD but not PPA so much. Neurotransmitters are the chemicals or hormones in your brain, such as serotonin, dopamine, and endorphins. Some atypical antidepressants include Effexor or Cymbalta.

Selective serotonin reuptake inhibitors are safely used for moms with PPA and PPD, even if they're breastfeeding. Serotonin regulates your mood, and this medication prevents the premature reabsorption of the hormone so you can benefit from the positive feelings. Moreover, this option has very few side effects. Names you may hear from your doctor are Zoloft, Prozac, or Paxil.

Finally, a doctor may try monoamine oxidase inhibitors (MOAs) or tricyclic antidepressants for PPD. These medications aren't commonly used because they take longer to work, and they can produce unwanted side effects. All antidepressants can cause side effects, but these two types can aggravate them. You may experience dry mouth, a lack of libido, fatigue, weight gain, restlessness, constipation, tremors, headaches, insomnia, or nausea. Discuss symptoms with your doctor if you want to change medications. The atypical or SSRI options may come with fewer side effects.

Most antidepressants take a few weeks to work, and you should take each dose, never skipping one. You might start with a small dose and increase it slowly by your doctor's orders. The most important thing with antidepressants or antianxiety medicine is that you must wean yourself off them slowly when you stop taking them. They can cause withdrawal symptoms if you stop abruptly. A doctor will supervise your weaning process, which may take a few weeks. Only start this process when your doctor gives you the green light, or you'll feel worse.

Hormone Therapy

Hormone therapy is a great option for moms suffering from PPD. According to research published by Massachusetts General Hospital and Harvard Medical School, hormone therapy can replace the plunge of estrogen after childbirth (2007). Your sudden drop in reproductive hormones after childbirth is likely responsible for your depression to some extent. The research included 23 moms with PPD who were treated with sublingual estradiol, which is a replacement hormone therapy for estrogen. Just two weeks later, 19 of the moms showed a remission of depression symptoms. All of the women initially had extremely low estrogen levels, even lower than women who suffer from gonadal failure. The female gonads are the ovaries. They produce eggs and hormones so that a failure would mean no production anymore. The results were a win for women who want to consider hormone replacement therapies to help them overcome PPD. Estrogen therapies are mostly reserved for women who suffer from estrogen deficiency, but it's something you may experience. Sometimes, it's also used with antidepressants.

Postpartum Psychosis Treatment

Postpartum psychosis is a serious condition, and it requires one or a combination of three medications. You may take antidepressants, mood stabilizers, and/or antipsychotic medicines to stabilize your moods and the chemical changes in your brain. If these medications can't stabilize your mood, you'll be recommended for electroconvulsive therapy. It sounds frightening, but it's a common way for doctors to use brief and highly tolerable electric pulses to trigger changes in your brain chemicals. It's a faster method of getting things done when medications aren't working well, and you don't need to fear it.

Moms who had postpartum psychosis will continue treatment after they leave the hospital, and this will be a combination of medication that tapers down over the coming weeks combined with therapy. Continued treatment is vital, especially if you have a personality disorder like bipolar or schizophrenia. Keep in mind that you can't wish a disorder away. Accept it, be compassionate enough toward yourself to seek treatment, and allow professionals to help you remain stable so you can enjoy motherhood.

No matter what condition you suffer from or how severe it became before you reached out, there's a treatment plan that could make your journey as enjoyable as you and your baby deserve. Remember to do your research to know what you want to discuss with your doctor, but being honest is the only way you can overcome PPD or PPA. Even milder issues may become more severe, so don't leave your mental health to improve on its own if your gut says otherwise. Continue your self-care at home, but be brave enough to ask for help. You won't be judged or ostracized if you take that priceless leap to seek medical help. It's what makes everyone see what a great mom you actually want to be. Additionally, don't forgo your self-care treatments if you're seeking professional help. The more you enhance your mental health, the better you'll be able to be anyone you choose, which in this case, may just be a great mom and partner.

CONCLUSION

Motherhood can be the most satisfying experience in life, or it can be the most daunting journey. The one you experience will be up to you now. The secrets of what comes after the birth of a child were revealed, and you know that your feelings aren't unusual. Your lack of interest in your new role is merely a sign of depression. Your inability to connect with your baby the way you dreamed about is simply a shadow of anxiety. You were overwhelmed and exhausted. Sure, no one can say being a new mom isn't exhausting, but is it normal to want to sleep all day but not be able to fall asleep? That just doesn't seem right. You might still experience the symptoms because neither PPD nor PPA will just vanish overnight. You may still have strange thoughts that make you worry, and you may continue to feel like you're not a good mother for some time. The void between what you now know and what you still feel will take time and effort to close.

Any mom who wonders whether she has the baby blues or full-blown PPD should consider her options to improve her mental health. Don't allow feelings of guilt and shame to prevent you from being the best mom you can be. Don't allow yourself to feel too emotionally tired to manage your newborn. Stay away from those sources that make you feel like you're a bad mother, and stop listening to people who say motherhood is a blissful journey without any worries and sadness. You're allowed to feel sad. You're allowed to be afraid for your baby's safety, but recognize when these feelings become something more. Having a baby isn't all rainbows and unicorns. Moms can even suffer from grief when the baby arrives, and it's normal for moms to doubt their abilities and instincts. The difference is that these feelings and thoughts shouldn't prevent you from caring for your baby or yourself.

Consider the logical side of becoming a mom. Just a few months ago, you felt independent, you could do what you wanted when you wanted to, you were financially secure, and you had a close connection with your partner. Heck, you probably wouldn't have planned a baby if you weren't close. In fairness, babies can also be unplanned, which will increase the stress, whether you have a partner or not. The moment you look at your baby, you know you feel a love like no other, even though disturbing thoughts and feelings sneak up on you. The fact that you're disturbed by them can be a good indicator that you haven't lost it, even if you think you will. Postpartum psychosis is also real, but it's rare, and you don't need to worry about it as long as you and/or your partner keeps a close eye on your symptoms.

Fear about the future can also wreak havoc on your mental health, and a baby, as much as you love them, can increase your fears because your family expands as soon as they arrive. You might be feeling the way you do if you lack social support as well. Maybe you have no family around, or your partner is always working long hours, leaving you to address your baby's needs when you're not even sure you can. There are so many reasons for postpartum mental health disorders, so never assume that you're immune to them. You could even show symptoms without realizing it. Learn to listen to your loved ones if they express concerns. Learn to ignore them if you feel depressed or anxious, and they tell you to stop being paranoid. Your gut is your number one friend in life. Always listen to it. You didn't read this book because you were just curious. You read it because you or a loved one is showing signs of mental health decline after having a baby.

You know what the differences are between the baby blues, PPD, PPA, postpartum psychosis, and even postpartum OCD now. Each condition is unique, and each one poses various problems that need to be addressed. You have a myriad of tools to do that now. You know how to care for yourself and your baby, even in moments of feeling hopeless and insecure. You know what to do when the most concerning symptoms arise, and more importantly, it's a great thing to know that every condition is treatable. You can still be the mother you want to be. You can still give your baby, partner, and yourself everything you deserve as a new family. The three self-care cornerstones will keep you and your baby in tip-top shape and lay the foundations of emotional resilience for the coming years. Mental health disorders are common in parents, and you know how much better your collective experience can be if you take care of them as soon as you notice them.

Get moving, eat the right foods that will replenish your body after having a baby, and take a moment to yourself when you need it. Use ancient tactics, proven to work by science, to become more than you can imagine. Elevate your mood in simple ways, none of which require hours away from your baby. If you need to, you can also take a break. Your partner is part of this amazing journey, and your friends may be more willing to help than you think. Allow the social lifeline to keep you going strong so nothing can derail you again. Part of your social network will be your partner, and you know how to keep things steady between you now. This is a time for the two of you to support each other, not break each other down or grow distant. You also have incredibly fun ways to bond with your baby to promote the type of relationship that sets the stage for your good mental health and their development.

You learned about the debate regarding breastfeeding. Who knew the answer was so simple? At the end of the day, I still urge you to seek professional help as soon as you feel overwhelmed or show signs of any postpartum disorder. All the tools you have *will* lay the resilience foundation, but asking for help is the best thing to do. There are so many professional treatments available should you need them. Again, I understand your pain, fears, and depression. As a mother and a therapist, I encourage you to navigate this journey with as many tools as you can, even if it must include medication and therapy. And if you should find this toolkit to be as helpful as I and many patients did, please leave a review where you can also let me know about your experience. I'd love to hear from you. A final word of advice would be that you take a moment to consider what the best thing for your family is right now. Determine what is in the best interest of you and your baby now, and take the first step to improvement, even if it's a small, wobbly step.

REFERENCES

Allen, K. (2015, March 9). *How long does PPD/A last?* Pacific Postpartum Support Society. https://postpartum.org/2015/03/long-ppda-last/

Barston, S. (n.d.). *Keeping your relationship strong during postpartum depression.* Seleni - Maternal Mental Health Institute. https://www.seleni.org/advice-support/2018/3/16/keeping-your-relationship-strong-during-postpartum-depression

Black, R. (2020, August 13). *Postpartum anxiety: Signs, symptoms, and treatments. Psycom.* https://www.psycom.net/postpartum-anxiety-postpartum-ocd

Brazier, Y., & Nwadike, V. R. (2019, November 5). *Postpartum depression: How long does it last?* Medical News Today. https://www.medicalnewstoday.com/articles/271217

Brusie, C., & Snyder, C. (2020, January 30). *Do you have these signs of postpartum OCD?* Verywell Family. https://www.verywellfamily. com/symptoms-of-postpartum-ocd-4083036

Buttner, M. M., Brock, R. L., O'Hara, M. W., & Stuart, S. (2015). Efficacy of yoga for depressed postpartum women: A randomized controlled trial. Complementary Therapies in Clinical Practice, 21(2), 94–100. https://doi.org/10.1016/j.ctcp.2015.03.003

Carberg, J., & Langdon, K. (2016). *Postpartum panic disorder.* Postpartum Depression. https://www.postpartumdepression.org/ postpartum-depression/types/panic-disorder/

Collno, S., & Fabian-Weber, N. (2020, February 10). *Postpartum anxiety: The other baby blues we need to talk about.* Parents. https://www.parents.com/parenting/moms/healthy-mom/the-other-postpartum-problem-anxiety/

De Bellefonds, C. (2018, May 29). *11 postpartum fitness tips for new moms.* What to Expect. https://www.whattoexpect.com/first-year/ postpartum/postpartum-fitness-tips/

Dellitt, J. (2018, January 17). *How exercise can help reduce postpartum depression.* Aaptiv. https://aaptiv.com/magazine/ exercise-reduce-postpartum-depression

Dennis, C.-L. (2003). *The effect of peer support on postpartum depression: A pilot randomized controlled trial.* The Canadian Journal of Psychiatry, 48(2), 115–124. https://doi.org/10. 1177/070674370304800209

Ellsworth-Bowers, E. R., & Corwin, E. J. (2012). *Nutrition and the psychoneuroimmunology of postpartum depression.* Nutrition Research Reviews, 25(1), 180–192. https://doi.org/10. 1017/s0954422412000091

Fairbrother, N., Janssen, P., Antony, M. M., Tucker, E., & Young, A. H. (2016). *Perinatal anxiety disorder prevalence and incidence.* Journal of Affective Disorders, 200, 148–155. https://doi.org/10. 1016/j.jad.2015.12.082

Fink, K. (2016, November 22). *10 mindfulness techniques for anxious moms, that all new moms should know.* Romper. https:// www.romper.com/p/10-mindfulness-techniques-for-anxious-moms-that-all-new-moms-should-know-22930

Garone, S., & Wallis, M. (2019, September 26). *Sleep consultants tell us how to survive the newborn days.* Healthline. https://www. healthline.com/health/sleep-consultants-share-tips-for-new-parents#The-Donts

Goyal, D., Gay, C., & Lee, K. (2009). *Fragmented maternal sleep is more strongly correlated with depressive symptoms than infant temperament at three months postpartum.* Archives of Women's Mental Health, 12(4), 229–237. https://doi.org/10.1007/s00737-009-0070-9

Green, L. (2021). *Is social media fuelling anxiety and depression among parents?* Priory Group. https://www.priorygroup.com/blog/is-social-media-fuelling-anxiety-and-depression-among-parents

Grimes, H. (2016, June 16). *How mindfulness protects against postpartum depression.* Mindful. https://www.mindful.org/ mindfulness-protects-post-partum-depression/

Hamdan, A., & Tamim, H. (2012). *The relationship between postpartum depression and breastfeeding.* The International Journal of Psychiatry in Medicine, 43(3), 243–259. https://doi.org/10. 2190/pm.43.3.d

Harvard Health Publishing. (2018, August 1). *How meditation helps with depression.* Harvard Health Publishing. https://www.health. harvard.edu/mind-and-mood/how-meditation-helps-with-depression

https://www.facebook.com/BountyClub. (2020, March 25). *Bonding with your baby.* Bounty. https://www.bounty.com/baby-0-to-12-months/postnatal-depression-and-bonding/bonding

Huber, R. B. (2014, March 27). *Four in 10 infants lack strong parental attachments.* Princeton University. https://www.princeton. edu/news/2014/03/27/four-10-infants-lack-strong-parental-attachments

Kelly, O., & Snyder, C. (2019). *Strange obsessions after birth can be due to postpartum OCD.* Verywell Mind. https://www. verywellmind.com/postpartum-obsessive-compulsive-disorder-2510665

Kleiman, K. (n.d.). *How to talk to your doctor about postpartum depression.* Seleni - Maternal Mental Health Institute. https://www.

seleni.org/advice-support/2018/3/16/how-to-talk-to-your-doctor-about-postpartum-depression

Ko, J. Y., Rockhill, K. M., Tong, V. T., Morrow, B., & Farr, S. L. (2017). *Trends in postpartum depressive symptoms — 27 states, 2004, 2008, and 2012.* MMWR. Morbidity and Mortality Weekly Report, 66(6), 153–158. https://doi.org/10.15585/mmwr.mm6606a1

Kripke, K. (2011, March 14). *How postpartum depression affects your marriage or partnership.* Postpartum Progress. https://postpartumprogress.com/how-postpartum-depression-affects-your-marriage-or-partnership

Kripke, K. (2013, March 21). *8 types of psychotherapy for PPD treatment.* Postpartum Progress. https://postpartumprogress.com/8-types-of-psychotherapy-for-postpartum-depression-treatment

Kubacky, G. (2013, May 2). *Active relaxation.* Gretchen Kubacky, Psy.D. http://drgretchenkubacky.com/thriving/active-relaxation/#.YMH5fb7ivIV

Landie, S. (2018, July 31). *Understand the difference between baby blues and postpartum depression.* Orlando Health. https://www.orlandohealth.com/content-hub/understand-the-difference-between-baby-blues-and-postpartum-depression

Massachusetts General Hospital. (2007, November 15). *Can estrogen be used to treat postpartum depression?* MGH Center for Women's Mental Health. https://womensmentalhealth.org/posts/estrogen-posptartum-depression/

Mauer, E. (2019, December 3). *A look at why relationships change after you have a baby.* Healthline. https://www.healthline.com/health/parenting/relationship-changes-after-baby#7.-Different-parenting-styles-can-add-extra-stress

Mayo Clinic Staff. (2018). *Postpartum depression - symptoms and causes.* Mayo Clinic; https://www.mayoclinic.org/diseases-conditions/postpartum-depression/symptoms-causes/syc-20376617

Mazel, S., & Lusskin, S. (2021, April 26). *12 signs of postpartum anxiety to look out for.* What to Expect. https://www.whattoexpect.com/first-year/postpartum-health-and-care/postpartum-anxiety/

MGH Center for Women's Mental Health. (2015, October 7). *Is it postpartum depression or postpartum anxiety? What's the difference?* MGH Center for Women's Mental Health. https://womensmentalhealth.org/posts/is-it-postpartum-depression-or-postpartum-anxiety-whats-the-difference/

Moran-Peters, J. A., Zauderer, C. R., Goldman, S., Baierlein, J., & Smith, A. E. (2014). *A quality improvement project focused on women's perceptions of skin-to-skin contact after cesarean birth.* Nursing for Women's Health, 18(4), 294–303. https://doi.org/10.1111/1751-486x.12135

National Childbirth Trust. (2021, January 20). *Pregnancy, parenthood and your social life.* National Childbirth Trust. https://www.nct.org.uk/life-parent/social-life-and-friendships/pregnancy-parenthood-and-your-social-life

National Health Institute. (2015, July 28). *Women's, men's brains respond differently to hungry infant's cries.* National Institutes of Health. https://www.nih.gov/news-events/news-releases/womens-mens-brains-respond-differently-hungry-infants-cries

National Health Services. (2018, December 13). *Sleep and tiredness after having a baby.* National Health Services. https://www.nhs.uk/conditions/baby/support-and-services/sleep-and-tiredness-after-having-a-baby/

National Health Services. (2020, December 7). *Keeping fit and healthy with a baby.* National Health Services. https://www.nhs.uk/conditions/baby/support-and-services/keeping-fit-and-healthy-with-a-baby/

Newsom, R. (2020, September 18). *Depression and sleep.* Sleep Foundation. https://www.sleepfoundation.org/mental-health/depression-and-sleep

Nichols, H., & Collier, J. (2017, November 7). *Postpartum depression: Tips for coping with it.* Medical News Today. https://www.medicalnewstoday.com/articles/320005#3.-Slowly-reintroduce-exercise

Ohio State University. (2014, November 19). *Research shows why antidepressants may be effective in postpartum depression.* Ohio State News. https://news.osu.edu/news/2014/11/19/research-shows-why-antidepressant-may-be-effective-in-postpartum-depression/

Pietrangelo, A., & Lay, J. (2016, December 7). *Postpartum depression: Symptoms, treatment, and more.* Healthline. https://www.healthline.com/health/depression/postpartum-depression#causes

Pinkowish, M. (2016, February 29). *How social support can help your postpartum depression.* Health. https://www.health.com/condition/depression/how-social-support-can-help-your-postpartum-depression

Poyatos-León, R., García-Hermoso, A., Sanabria-Martínez, G., Álvarez-Bueno, C., Cavero-Redondo, I., & Martínez-Vizcaíno, V. (2017). *Effects of exercise-based interventions on postpartum depression: A meta-analysis of randomized controlled trials.* Birth, 44(3), 200–208. https://doi.org/10.1111/birt.12294

Rios, A. C., Maurya, P. K., Pedrini, M., Zeni-Graiff, M., Asevedo, E., Mansur, R. B., Wieck, A., Grassi-Oliveira, R., McIntyre, R. S., Hayashi, M. A. F., & Brietzke, E. (2017). *Microbiota abnormalities and the therapeutic potential of probiotics in the treatment of mood disorders.* Reviews in the Neurosciences, 28(7). https://doi.org/10.1515/revneuro-2017-0001

Robinson, L. (2020, October). *Building a secure attachment bond with your baby.* Help Guide. https://www.helpguide.org/articles/parenting-family/building-a-secure-attachment-bond-with-your-baby.htm#

Sit, D. K. Y., & Wisner, K. L. (2009). *Identification of postpartum depression.* Clinical Obstetrics and Gynecology, 52(3), 456–468. https://doi.org/10.1097/grf.0b013e3181b5a57c

Smith, M., Segal, J., & Glezer, A. (2019). *Postpartum depression and the baby blues.* Help Guide. https://www.helpguide.org/articles/depression/postpartum-depression-and-the-baby-blues.htm

Smith, R. (2014, May 21). *Depression affects mothers most when a child is four years old.* The Telegraph. https://www.telegraph.co.uk/women/womens-health/10843213/Depression-affects-mothers-most-when-child-is-four-years-old.html

Sokol, R. (2020, February 12). *How to stay social when you're a new parent.* Family Education. https://www.familyeducation.com/adjusting-new-motherhood/how-to-stay-social-when-youre-a-new-parent

Stone, K. (2016, August 30). *Postpartum depression and social media: 6 things you need to know.* Postpartum Progress. https://postpartumprogress.com/postpartum-depression-and-social-media

Stygar, K., & Zadroga, J. (2021, April 20). *Infants have mental health needs, too.* Mayo Clinic Health System. https://www.mayoclinichealthsystem.org/hometown-health/speaking-of-health/infants-have-mental-health-needs-too

Sumner, C. (2005, October 3). *8 marriage issues you'll face after baby and how to solve them.* Parents. https://www.parents.com/parenting/relationships/staying-close/marriage-after-baby/

Suni, E. (2020, December 10). *Anxiety and sleep.* Sleep Foundation. https://www.sleepfoundation.org/mental-health/anxiety-and-sleep

Surkan, P. J., Peterson, K. E., Hughes, M. D., & Gottlieb, B. R. (2006). *The role of social networks and support in postpartum women's depression: A multiethnic urban sample.* Maternal and Child Health Journal, 10(4), 375–383. https://doi.org/10.1007/s10995-005-0056-9

Tallents, C. (2018, April 10). *5 foods to fight postpartum depression.* Motherly. https://www.mother.ly/lifestyle/5-foods-to-help-keep-postpartum-depression-at-bay

Taylor, M. (2020, June 30). *Facts on SIDS.* What to Expect. https://www.whattoexpect.com/first-year/sids.aspx

U.S. Department of Health and Human Services. (2018, October 18). *Postpartum depression.* Women's Health. https://www.womenshealth.gov/mental-health/mental-health-conditions/postpartum-depression

Wiener, L. (2007, October 24). *Stressed? 28 ways to unwind - by tonight.* Parents. https://www.parents.com/baby/new-parent/emotions/ways-to-unwind/?slide=slide_83e3b031-df0a-4aa0-9b83-05f385bafad4#

Wisner, W., & Snyder, C. (2020, July 6). *Do I have postpartum blues or postpartum depression?* Verywell Family. https://www.verywellfamily.com/postpartum-blues-vs-postpartum-depression-4770580

Zander-Schellenberg, T., Collins, I. M., Miché, M., Guttmann, C., Lieb, R., & Wahl, K. (2020). *Does laughing have a stress-buffering effect in daily life? An intensive longitudinal study.* Plos One, 15(7), e0235851. https://doi.org/10.1371/journal.pone.0235851

IMAGE REFERENCES

Image One. (n.d.). In Pixabay. https://pixabay.com/photos/baby-mother-infant-child-female-821625/

Image Two. (n.d.). In Pixabay. https://pixabay.com/photos/ad-baby-baby-photography-small-2946440/

Image Three. (n.d.). In Pixabay. https://pixabay.com/photos/baby-feet-baby-feet-ten-small-1595389/

Image Four. (n.d.). In Pixabay. https://pixabay.com/photos/newborn-infant-baby-mother-2186612/

Image Five. (n.d.). In Pixabay. https://pixabay.com/photos/baby-flying-floating-happy-sky-2545745/

Image Six. (n.d.). In Pixabay. https://pixabay.com/photos/small-child-swim-wash-baby-infant-788006/

Image Seven. (n.d.). In Pixabay. https://pixabay.com/photos/mom-spacer-maternity-education-5088669/

Image Eight. (n.d.). In Pixabay. https://pixabay.com/photos/grilled-chicken-quinoa-salad-1334632/

Image Nine. (n.d.). In Pixabay. https://pixabay.com/photos/infant-newborn-love-baby-son-4025284/

Image Ten. (n.d.). In Pixabay. https://pixabay.com/photos/bath-foam-girl-relax-spa-frothy-5509230/

Image Eleven. (n.d.). In Pixabay. https://pixabay.com/photos/baby-bottle-suck-feed-mother-105063/

Image Twelve. (n.d.). In Pixabay. https://pixabay.com/photos/people-leisure-tree-lifestyle-3250299/

Image Thirteen. (n.d.). In Pixabay. https://pixabay.com/photos/people-baby-blanket-boy-child-2942977/

Image Fourteen. (n.d.). In Pixabay. https://pixabay.com/photos/friends-girls-best-friends-women-842580/

Image Fifteen. (n.d.). In Pixabay. https://pixabay.com/photos/people-holding-hands-sunset-man-2561053/

Image Sixteen. (n.d.). In Pixabay. https://pixabay.com/photos/family-newborn-baby-child-infant-2610205/

Image Seventeen. (n.d.). In Pixabay. https://pixabay.com/photos/father-baby-portrait-infant-22194/

Image Eighteen. (n.d.). In Pixabay. https://pixabay.com/photos/baby-flowers-in-her-hair-hairband-1232243/

Image Nineteen. (n.d.). In Pixabay. https://pixabay.com/photos/baby-newborn-child-parenting-4100420/

Image Twenty. (n.d.). In Pixabay. https://pixabay.com/photos/psychologist-psychoanalyst-girl-6008048/

Made in the USA
Coppell, TX
18 September 2022

83311254R00083